Moments of Truth, Gifts of Love

WOMEN OF COMMUNITY AND SPIRIT
JOURNEY THROUGH BREAST CANCER

"In the past 75 years, thanks to improvements in diagnosis and treatment, the death rate due to breast cancer has dropped from 50% to 15%. How wonderful it is to read the compelling stories written by these courageous survivors!"

Dr. Wende Logan-Young
Elizabeth Wende Breast Care, LLC
www.ewbc.com

"If Madeleine Albright is right about that special place in hell for women who do not help other women, then the spiritual corollary is also true. There's a special place in heaven for women who help other women. With this book, Eve Strella reaches out to women who are facing breast cancer, women who have survived it, and women who know other women in either category. Like Eve herself, this collection is warm, funny, and filled with hope. It will make you laugh. It will make you cry. And, it will make you fundamentally, powerfully, aware of what it means to be a woman who faces this dreaded illness with spunk and bravery and an appreciation for joy."

Dr. Marlene Caroselli
author, corporate trainer, and keynote speaker
mccpd@frontiernet.net

W9-BDN-061

"Each of the authors shares a unique perspective on her challenges with breast cancer. I hope the readers, whether patient or family, discover the strength within these stories, within themselves, and, as importantly, come to realize that they are not alone on their journey."

Jan Dombrowski, M.D.
Medical Director, Pluta Cancer Center, Rochester New York

"Many of us have been affected by cancer. We have either had cancer, someone we love has it, or it has caused us to lose someone we treasure. Deeply sharing with us, the authors in these profound and moving stories guide us through their honest journeys of understanding what it means "to live through cancer." To be our most compassionate selves here on earth, we need to listen."

Terry Laszlo-Gopadze
Cancer survivor and creator of The Spirit of a Woman:
Stories to Empower and Inspire
www.womens-spirit.com

"Very touching and sensitive stories. They give such insight and encouragement and help one to embrace life to its fullest each and every day. Most importantly, know that as a cancer patient, you are a survivor from the day you are diagnosed."

Gail Ferris-Cowie, RNOCN
Nurse Manager, Pluta Cancer Center
Rochester, New York

"*Moments of Truth, Gifts of Love: Women of Community and Spirit Journey through Breast Cancer* is a heartwarming collection of scathingly truthful and powerfully mesmerizing stories told by a community of women in their own strong voices. Though breast cancer is a challenging disease that does not always end up pretty and pink and is not always won, this book chalks one up for the sisterhood."

Holly Anderson
Executive Director
Breast Cancer Coalition of Rochester
holly@bccr.org
www.bccr.org
www.breastcancercoalition.org
United Way Donor Choice #2334

"It has been 15 years since I met and cared for my first patient with a brain tumor. His wife was a nurse in our Operating Room. He worked as a nurse in the prison system. During the 2 years he fought his cancer, he sought out the most aggressive treatment, hoping to spend more time with his children. I am often asked how I deal with all the tragedy associated with cancer. My answer is easy. Patients and their families show so much courage; it is very inspiring."

Every day is a gift; that is why it is called the present.

Susan O. Smith, Adult Nurse Practitioner
University of Rochester
Rochester, New York

Moments of Truth, Gifts of Love

Contributors:

Linda Allen

Judi Baronsky

Pat Battaglia

Pat Bernhard

Theresa Bronte

Andrea Caruso

Barbara Compa

Alison Currie

Myra Morgan, M.D.

Linda Morreale

Eve Strella-Ribson

Laura Robertaccio

Wendy White-Ryan, M.D.

Margaret Schuler

Janet Stager

Bonnie Thies

Jane Vallely

Mary Ellen Vollmer

Judy Wood

Moments of Truth, Gifts of Love

WOMEN OF COMMUNITY AND SPIRIT
JOURNEY THROUGH BREAST CANCER

EVE STRELLA-RIBSON
BOOK ORGANIZER / CREATOR / CONTRIBUTOR

PRODUCTIVITY PUBLICATIONS
ROCHESTER, NEW YORK

ISBN: 978-0-9729119-7-9

Published by Productivity Publications, Rochester, New York
http://www.productivitypublications.com

Cover by Sarah Page, SMP Studios, http://www.smpstudios.com/

Cover photography by Eve Strella-Ribson
http://www.strellaandassociates.com, estrella@strellaandassociates.com

Photos of Eve Strella-Ribson by Bob Brown, rbrown1973@googlemail.com

Arimidex® and Faslodex® are registered trademarks of AstraZeneca Global

Adriamycin® and Aromasin® are registered trademarks of Pfizer

Benadryl® is a registered trademark of Johnson and Johnson

Cipro® is a registered trademark of Bayer Healthcare Pharmaceuticals

Cytoxan®, Ixempra®, Taxol® are registered trademarks of Bristol-Myers Squibb

Herceptin® is a registered trademark of Genentech, Inc.

Neosporin® is a registered trademark of Warner-Lambert Company, LLC

Neulasta® is a registered trademark of Amgen, Inc.

OxyContin® is a registered trademark of Purdue Pharma L.P.

Taxotere® is a registered trademark of Aventis Pharma S.a.

Xeloda® is a registered trademark of Hoffman-LaRoche Inc.

Dedication

I dedicate this book to my husband Edward J. Ribson, who has been by my side every step without complaint, always supportive, giving me love, hope, and laughter.

I am so lucky to have you in my life … I love you Eddie.

BOOKS TO WHICH EVE STRELLA-RIBSON HAS CONTRIBUTED

The Spirit of a Woman: Stories to Empower and Inspire
Edited by Terry Laszlo-Gopadze www.womens-spirit.com

*Quality Care: Prescriptions for Injecting Quality
into Healthcare Systems*
Marlene Caroselli, Ed.D. with Linda Edison

50 Activities for Promoting Ethics in the Organization
Marlene Caroselli, Ed.D.

Jan's Rainbow
Lindsay Collier

Defining Moments
Edited by Susan Rae Baker

Table of Contents

Foreword

BY EDWARD J. RIBSON

It was the first time I knew something was definitely wrong. For the past couple of weeks, each morning before leaving for work, I had been asking my wife to see a doctor about the headaches and dizziness she had been experiencing. I did not really think that anything was seriously amiss with Eve, but I didn't want to take chances with the most important person in my life. But now, on a quiet May evening, I was more than a little worried.

I had been out in our private observatory, Stardust. Since the summer of 2004 when Eve and I had built Stardust, we had spent many clear nights exploring the heavens together. As we each peered into the telescope eyepiece, we often felt transported away from our mundane suburban surroundings. Like shipmates and soul mates sailing the cosmic sea of time and space, we wanted to experience as much of the universe as possible over the course of a lifetime. Our journey together was both cosmic and spiritual, and the observatory became a sacred place that would bind us even more closely. In many respects, evenings together in Stardust illuminated our love, not only for the cosmos, but also for each other.

On this particular evening, I rotated the observatory dome so that the constellation of Hercules was visible as it slowly arced toward the zenith and set the telescope computer to aim the scope at M13 in Hercules, the most spectacular globular star cluster visible from the northern hemisphere. Globular star clusters form a galactic halo as they orbit the spiral disc of our Milky Way galaxy like bees swarming about an enormous dish-shaped luminous hive. I watched as the red LEDs on the computer readout went to zero, at which point the telescope was aimed at M13. Barely visible to the unaided eye, M13 appeared through the scope as a blazing ball of stars—about 300,000 if one could take time to count them all. Light takes an entire century to travel from one side of M13 to the other and more than 25,000 years to travel from M13 to Earth.

The mind can reel with a sense of insignificance from contemplating such distances. But that night, the most precious person in my life—in this universe or in any other—was back in the house, less than 100 feet away. Suddenly, I felt a pang of loneliness bordering on dread, as though that 100-foot separation spanned an entire galaxy. I trotted back to the house to find Eve sitting at her computer. She looked wearied and fatigued. When I asked whether she wanted to take a look at M13 before I closed up the observatory, she told me that she had been vomiting that day and didn't have the energy to do much of anything. Something was wrong. I didn't know what, but something was definitely wrong. Again, I told her that she needed to see her doctor, and, for the first time, she agreed.

Eve's physician sent her for an MRI scan, and the next day she learned that a tumor was pressing against her brain stem. As bad as that was, we were determined to deal with it. Worse news followed a PET scan in early June. Eve and I had been watching television in the living room when the phone rang. Eve put the phone on speaker. I listened to the quiet voice of her oncologist as he told her that the scan had revealed cancerous lesions in her lungs and on a lymph node. He told Eve that it had probably metastasized from the triple negative breast cancer for which she had received chemotherapy and radiation therapy in 2007. I think I stopped breathing for several moments. Even though Eve and I were well aware of the possibility of a recurrence of triple negative breast cancer, we had determined to be optimistic.

An image flashed into my mind from our vacation in Hawaii seven months earlier. Eve and I had gone down to the ocean by our hotel to bounce in the waves. I entered the water first. Surf was surging high on the beach as waves came in fast and hard. A big one lifted me vertically a few feet. Hoping that Eve had already entered the water, I turned to look back. To my shock, she was hesitating in ankle-deep surf when she saw the wave coming. At the last instant, she turned to race back up onto the beach, but it was too late. The same wave that had lifted me slammed her from behind with terrific force, knocking her down.

As the water retreated, Eve was left rolling in sandy surf, unable to regain her footing or to get to deeper water. The wave had torn Eve's prescription sunglasses off, and I saw a look of helpless terror in her eyes. Knowing, as Eve and I did, that eleven people had recently drowned in the waters off Kauai (two of them women who had simply been strolling along a beach when they were hit by a sudden wave and washed out to sea) was not reassuring! As a second wave lifted me, I seemed to be looking down on Eve from a surreal height. I shouted her name to let her know that I saw her and was coming as quickly as possible, but getting out of the water proved nearly as difficult for me as getting in had been for her. The second wave struck Eve with full force while she was on her hands and knees. The surge washed her up toward the beach and then pulled her rolling back out to where the waves were breaking. As I struggled to reach her, I had never felt so helpless and scared. Luckily, a passer-by on the beach helped Eve out of the water before a third big wave arrived. (To my amazement, after a few minutes, Eve decided to go right back in the water—this time successfully!)

A similar feeling of terrified helplessness, only more intense, swept over me as I sat listening to Eve's oncologist tell us in carefully chosen words that the cancer could not be cured but would be very manageable over the period of survivability. For a moment, I asked myself if this was a nightmare. I hugged Eve's legs and sobbed, telling her (not for the first or last time) that I would never let her go.

I will not attempt to recount Eve's battle with cancer here. Later in this book, Eve tells her story far better than I ever could. However, I will mention some of the ways in which Eve's battle has changed my spiritual outlook and heightened my awareness of what I can only describe as a previously unsuspected universe of people.

Summer 2009 was not a season Eve and I would ever care to relive. Shortly after brain surgery, Eve began several rounds of full brain radiation to be followed by an indeterminate number of rounds of chemotherapy. One day in July, I had been feeling especially gloomy at work. Suddenly, my head ached as though someone had rammed a blunt steel rod through my left temple and out the back of my skull. I choked back tears while driving home that evening. I was determined that Eve not see me in that condition, but, in spite of myself, when I got home and hugged Eve, I broke down again. Mentally cussing myself, I told Eve that I was just a little depressed and went upstairs to my study. I realized that I would have to get past that sort of depression. Not only was it not good for Eve, it was threatening to incapacitate me. I eventually got past it by putting the future out of my head and living in the moment. I had come to realize what I think Eve had long since discovered: you cannot function with a constant sense of impending doom.

Living in the moment was not something that I did consciously or purposely. It just happened. Initially, I was not even aware of the change, except that my terrific headaches had stopped. I had learned to be happy again—or at least not too sad—by living in the moment.

I also started praying a lot. I don't say that in a sanctimonious way because, for most of my life, I have wavered between pantheism and atheism. I do not buy into the concept of a God who reveals Himself only to a few prophets and shamans who have come down from mountaintops and out of deserts to announce to the rest of us that they have had some sort of privileged epiphany. If God exists, His presence would be felt by all of us, not just by a select few who claim to have spoken with God and who insist that we believe in their teachings. God's existence or non-existence is independent of our beliefs. However, it is also possible that we each experience God on our own without recognizing the experience for what it actually is. So while my faith may be weak, my hope is great that Someone out there is hearing my prayers. Quite possibly, many of them have already been answered.

I have also come to realize that two of life's most priceless gifts are health and time. Given good health and sufficient time, we can achieve whatever else we desire. Since none of us knows how much time and good health we have left, these gifts ought not to be squandered.

Ever since Eve had started undergoing treatment, she and I have grown increasingly aware of another of life's most precious gifts—the people around us: the medical professionals, family, friends, and neighbors who have supported and continue to support Eve (and me) throughout this battle. Most astounding to me, though, have been those who were initially strangers—people who, perhaps noticing Eve's bald head, have come up to her and introduced themselves at supermarkets, restaurants, concerts, and other public events as breast cancer patients.

A couple of summers ago, Eve and I attended a Pat Benatar/ Blondie concert with friends at CMAC, the Finger Lakes open-air performing arts center. During the intermission, two young ladies came down from their seats behind us and introduced themselves to Eve. I believe they were in their late twenties or early thirties, but they both appeared so young and vibrant that I initially assumed they were not much older than twenty. They had noticed that Eve was bald under her signature baseball cap. I consciously had to keep my jaw from dropping open in disbelief when they both revealed themselves as breast cancer patients. When they mentioned to Eve that they both had ports installed for blood work and chemo infusions, I noticed the tubes running just beneath the skin along the sides of their necks. The husband of one of the young women chatted with me and offered much reassurance. I do hope God exists, because I need someone to thank for putting Eve and me on the same planet with each other and with such wonderful people! Before Eve had been diagnosed, we had hardly ever given a thought to the prevalence of breast cancer. Now we encounter breast cancer warriors almost everywhere.

All too often, scientific knowledge can leave us feeling small and insignificant. If we were to gaze back 25,000 light-years in earth's direction from M13, our sun would not be evident among the two hundred billion other stars in the Milky Way galaxy's spiral disc, not even if we had the most powerful telescopes currently on earth at our disposal. Yet, here on earth, Eve and I have become aware of another universe—a universe of breast cancer warriors and survivors. And each of their spirits holds a cosmos of experiences within. This book is an introduction to that universe.

MY BIO

Edward Ribson holds a Bachelor of Science degree in biology and is currently employed as a public health official in the Division of Environmental Health at a county health department. His avocations are astronomy and astrophysics. His other interests range from art and art history to Greek Bronze Age prehistory, Greek mythology, classical literature, and the early history of Christianity. Mr. Ribson holds memberships in the Astronomy Section of the Rochester Academy of Science and in the International Dark-Sky Association.

Acknowledgments

"If trouble hearing Angels song with thine ears, try listening with thy heart." Meriel Stelliger

This book would not have been possible without the contributors who shared their stories: Linda Allen, Judith Baronsky, Pat Battaglia, Pat Bernhard, Theresa Bronte, Andrea Caruso, Barbara Compa, Alison Currie, Myra Morgan, M.D., Linda Morreale, Laura Robertaccio, Wendy White-Ryan, M.D., Margaret Schuler, Janet Stager, Bonnie Thies, Jane Vallely, Mary Ellen Vollmer, and Judy Wood. I thank each and every one of them from the bottom of my heart.

My husband Ed has been an exceptional support throughout this process. He is my knight in shining armor and my guiding star. As my editor, he polishes my words until they shine. When I asked him to discuss his own spiritual odyssey since my diagnosis in a foreword for this book, he was reluctant at first to make public his personal thoughts and emotions, but I thought that his experience as a spouse would offer readers a rare perspective, and it has indeed. I love waking up next to you every morning, Eddie. I love you.

My sister Kareen lives in New Jersey and has not been able to travel to my home in Pittsford, New York since my cancer returned, but we still talk at least once a week. I update her on my health, the book, and life in general, and she showers me with encouragement and love. I am very lucky to have her in my life. She is my cheerleader for all my endeavors. Kareen wrote the wonderful story on a sister's love and support for this book. Thanks, Sis.

A special thank you goes to my book editor, publisher, and good friend, Kay Whipple. I am so grateful for her many gifts and incredible talent. Her knowledge of publishing, editing, and analyzing flow was a godsend. She guided the direction of this book and helped me to understand the complexities of publishing. I thank her for her patience throughout this process.

My good friend and mentor, Dr. Marlene Caroselli, has guided me and shared her wisdom and experience every step of the way. She brings me goodie baskets filled with really cool items. It has been endless fun unwrapping everything. I often laugh, wondering how she delivers baskets to the front porch without being seen. She keeps me smiling by e-mailing me jokes nearly every day. Thank you for all you do, Marlene.

I am so grateful to have Sarah Page on board as my graphic artist. She designed a book cover that took my breath away. I sent her a photograph that I took looking down the lane from the farm where I was raised in Western Pennsylvania. She took that photo and magically transformed it. I wanted the lane to represent "the Journey," and that it does. Thank you, Sarah.

I give thanks to my late father, Robert M. Johnston, Sr., for all the gifts he gave me over the course of a lifetime. My father suffered from multiple cancers and died in his favorite chair in the living room of the house we helped him build. Our family surrounded him with a circle of love during his final days. I miss you so much, Dad.

I can't thank my late husband, David Owen Strella, enough for all he has done for me. I am the person I am today because of his love, support, guidance, patience, hugs, and kisses. He opened the world for me by giving me confidence to tackle anything that got in my way. He helped me grow continually and expanded my vision in every venture I took on. David watched over me every day and continues to do so in spirit. David, I thank you for EVERYTHING!

I also want to thank my beloved kittens, Kirk and Burt, for their unconditional love and affection. These little pussycat brothers keep me entertained and laughing. As I look over the side of my desk, I see them lying side by side—often in the oddest positions—wrapped sound asleep in each other's love. Thank you, boys.

Introduction

BY EVE STRELLA-RIBSON & EDWARD J. RIBSON

"There are in the end three things that last: Faith, Hope and Love, and the greatest of these is Love."
Paul, Corinthians 13:13

The National Cancer Institute has reported that an estimated 207,090 women and 1,970 men would develop breast cancer in the USA in 2010. For nearly 40,000 women and 400 men, the disease will prove fatal. Of the women diagnosed with breast cancer, nearly 90 percent are expected to survive at least five years. Compared to the historical 75 percent survival rate, this comes as good news, but for those recently diagnosed with breast cancer, it is far from good enough. Our minds tend to go numb when we contemplate the nearly 210,000 individuals expected to develop the disease in a single year in the USA alone, and we fail to see the faces of the individuals behind such figures. By focusing on the stories of nineteen women diagnosed with breast cancer in upstate New York, this book attempts to put a human face on the statistics. For anyone recently diagnosed with breast cancer, this book's message is simple: You are not alone. And you are not just a statistic.

The contributors to this book have families, homes, and gardens. They vacation, hike, climb mountains, dive in the ocean, and run marathons. They take enormous pride in their children and grandchildren. Each contributor is a unique individual, but each also belongs to what may be regarded as a sisterhood of breast cancer patients—a sorority none ever sought to join. No pledge was required for involuntary membership in this sorority. The only initiation was a positive diagnosis of cancer, when in less than a heartbeat, life was set reeling on edge or turned upside down. Dreams and aspirations for the future were instantly put on hold as the new reality replaced each woman's former life with shadowy uncertainties.

Although each woman has her own unique story to tell, the common threads of faith, hope, and love run throughout these stories. Faith, hope, and love are the cardinal virtues cited by St. Paul in his Letter to the Church in Corinth. However, these virtues transcend any single religion or place of worship.

Faith offers a personal connection to a higher power. For some, a breast cancer diagnosis is the catalyst for a more entrenched and meaningful relationship with the Divine. For others, a breast cancer diagnosis is so life-shaking that their relationship with God is renewed and confirmed. Many who had never before held God in their hearts now find Him within themselves, in others, and in the world beyond. Faith changes our perception of the world. Sunrises and sunsets are no longer merely routine events that occur as our planet rotates. Seen though new eyes, these events and the days whose arrival and departure they herald are now sources of wonder and appreciation.

As Ruth Ann Schabacker once said, *"Each day comes bearing its own gifts. Untie the ribbons."* So, faith is a gift that reveals the other gifts that lie before us as well: renewed spiritual insight and a heightened appreciation of all that is around and beyond us.

As the second cardinal virtue, hope is also a common thread joining these stories. We hope for things both great and small. We hope for a cure, to be able to watch our children grow, to have our health and vitality back. We hope to be able to taste food again and to have our hair back! We hope for a future of possibilities. In the words of William Sloane Coffin Jr., "*Hope arouses, as nothing else can arouse, a passion for the possible.*"

Love is the third and greatest cardinal virtue. Its thread binds not only these stories but their contributors as well. Love is potentially all-encompassing in its scope and limitless in its passion or strength. We may love nature, the visible cosmos, and we may love the unseen force, power, or principle from whence that universe sprang into existence. We may worship God as that creative force, power, or principle. If we love God and His handiwork, then it follows that we should love each other and ourselves as well, for we are all part of God's creation, part of the cosmos. We are, in fact, that part of the universe that has evolved a consciousness capable of gazing out on itself and contemplating its wonders. And, as we go through life, our individual experiences form a personal universe within each of us. How sad it is that it sometimes takes a potentially fatal disease like cancer to make us aware of our significance in the creation and of our significance to each other! However that awareness comes to us, love is a gift of Spirit to be embraced. Since our days in this world are limited— none of us knows how much time remains to us—our love should be limitless. We need to love life and to love our families, friends, and all those who support us (caregivers, medical teams, chemo nurses, and many others) as if each day was our last. Without our support system, we would not have a chance at battling this disease and moving, once again, out into the world.

This book is divided into five sections. *The Loving Spirit* focuses on love, the gift that forms an unbreakable bond between breast cancer patients and their families and friends. *The Human Spirit* focuses on hope, the gift that motivates breast cancer fighters even during the worst days of chemo and radiation therapy. This section has to do with what we're made of and hope is a part of that equation. *The Holy Spirit* focuses on faith, the gift that enables breast cancer warriors to bond with a higher power in the battle against this disease. *The Changing Spirit* focuses on the evolving spiritual transformation of breast cancer patients and of those who love and support them. This division, of course, is somewhat arbitrary since many of the stories illuminate more than just one gift of Spirit. The last section, *The Family Spirit,* demonstrates the special gift of a sister's love, and highlights the thoughts and experiences of those who support cancer patients.

As of this writing, one of this book's contributors has passed on. The rest continue the battle either to regain their former lives or to forge new lives. As members in the community of breast cancer survivors, they support and pray for one another and those who come after them, sisters in faith, hope, and love. Here then are their stories to enlighten and inspire us, to fill us occasionally with laughter and tears, and, above all, to let readers know: *You are not alone.*

Section One:
The Loving Spirit

Families and friends who love and support us through life's difficult journeys are the greatest blessings along the path. Sometimes we don't realize how much we are loved until life's traumas shine a light on these people who are life's greatest gifts.

"A real friend knows when to listen, when to stop listening, when to talk, when to stop talking, when to pour wine, and when to stop pouring and just hand over the bottle."

LEE FRANKLIN

"A friend is a person with whom you dare to be yourself."

FRANK CRANE

"Your friend is the man who knows all about you, and still likes you."

ELBERT HUBBARD

$$\textbf{1}$$

Impressions of a Journey

BY BARBARA OERTEL COMPA

"Remember, no matter where you go, there you are!"
Confucius

MY DIAGNOSIS:

On June 11, 2008, a needle biopsy confirmed a diagnosis of invasive ductal carcinoma of my left breast. I was 57 years old. The tumor was approximately 2x3.9 cm, nuclear grade 2, estrogen and progesterone positive. The surgeon suggested a partial mastectomy followed by a new form of radiation in which a balloon was inserted where the tumor had been. It would be loaded with seeds of radiation twice a day for five days. After the surgery on July 21, 2008, however, the margins were found not to be clear, and cancer cells were found in seven of the nineteen lymph nodes. I began six rounds of chemo (TAC), followed by a left mastectomy, and seven weeks of radiation five times a week. On June 11, 2009, I had surgery again to rebuild the left breast, followed by reduction of both breasts in January 2010. A nipple was added in April 2010, and the final tattooing was in August. I will be taking Arimidex daily for five years to block the hormones which fed my cancer.

MY JOURNEY:

The lights were dimmed in the room after the mammogram, and the nurse folded linens and re-arranged papers without speaking or looking at me. A doctor came through the door quickly, in a state of panic, poor guy.

"There is a large area in there…"

I replied that I was always called back because I am dense (hopefully not in reference to my brain).

"It's a mass in there."

He was visibly upset. Doom and gloom. He was probably surprised when I laughed. I had been feeling a lump. It had been confirmed by my GYN, who had sent me for the test, so obviously I was aware. What he didn't know was the level of disorganization permeating my life. I thought he had said, "It's a mess in there," and was visualizing the tangle of veins and ducts and whatever, which resembled my workroom/storage room at home: "the land of unrealized dreams" that was the story of my life. It struck me as funny, and it wasn't until after a few months (while talking to my boss, who had sent me to organization workshops) that I realized he had actually said "mass." Oh well.

The room in which the diagnosis was confirmed was bright and warm, decorated with the doctor's family photos and grandchildren's drawings. It didn't even look like an examining room. The doctor was an incredibly beautiful woman with her white hair in a loose Victorian-era bun. Seeing her was a treat in itself, and I felt like I was under a spell. The diagnosis was clear-cut and matter-of-fact. I felt so well cared for from the first moment—a passenger on a classy "breast cancer express" which would take me on a tour of myself.

ANGELS COME IN DIFFERENT PACKAGES

I don't use the term "angels" lightly. It takes a gut feeling to know if a person actually qualifies as an angel in my life, and most people are unaware of their status and would even deny it. They are at the right place at the right time when needed, despite what their intentions are.

My first angel was a friend who had been diagnosed with uterine cancer. She had surgery, was receiving treatment, and was my first peer with cancer. I was trying to be there for her, but felt awkward with the thought of the magnitude of "the diagnosis" for a person with young children. We were talking about her hysterectomy and issues of menopause, and I mentioned that I had not even thought about seeing my gynecologist for several years, since I had retired. She said with an authority that made me take notice, "Do it NOW." I made the appointment.

The second encounter came on that endless dark time after diagnosis. It seemed like a month, but it was only the next day. I needed support but wanted to control when and how I would get it. I wanted anonymity and information. I Googled "online breast cancer support" and got just what I needed. Who would have thought there were angels in cyberspace? Two wonderful young women actually paid for and ran a site for survivors. They researched issues and created a safe place for us to come to terms with our issues and meet others. They had "meet-ups," and I went to my first one at a coffee shop. This is how naïve I was: I was looking for a group of bald women! I had no idea the support would continue for years after treatment. I learned that I was a warrior from the day I was diagnosed, and I immediately felt part of the sisterhood that would be my constant support from then on.

I have worked with people with disabilities my whole adult life, so I am familiar with illness, surgeries, and physical limitations. What I didn't realize is the number of people who have been through the invisible disease I was about to experience. People I have known forever seemed to pop into my life, having gone through this in one way or another. Their experiences helped me through my own. People share when they feel it will help others. I hope that goes for me as well. Now that I am no longer "cancer girl," I think of myself as normal—to remember the experience in such a way that it doesn't permeate my life. I won't give it that power.

PARTY TIME!

My favorite angel encounters came from my own family. On my confirmation day, my twenty-four-year-old daughter Corey was with me. "You have been with me during all my medical appointments, and I will be here with you."

The doctor asked me if I wanted her to talk to my daughter, and I said, "No, she would probably freak out."

When I went out to the waiting room for a break, she had organized a party atmosphere with the men whose wives were having their own party in the inner sanctum. One of her new friends was out getting coffee for her, and she had discovered her former elementary school principal, who was there with her mother. I had been deliberating how to break the news, but with a smile on everyone's face and music in the air, I was just able to blurt it out without anyone even noticing.

From that moment on, Corey was unflappable. She became my press agent and my cheerleader. When the phone rang in the car on the way home, she broke the news to her stoic twenty-one-year-old brother Rob, who cried while walking around Boston talking on his cell. Go figure! Since he was freaking out, I figured I'd better get to my husband before Rob did, so I called and caught him just as he was about to walk into his own retirement party after 15 years on the job. I really know how to make a party fun for a guy! Angel Larry has been here for me every minute of every day and is back to work at a new job.

The third angel materialized in the form of Rob, who surprised me by organizing a huge music party and fund-raiser here in Rochester, New York. His band from Boston and three other bands (including Larry's) raised $2000 for the cause. Most of us have love and support from all our friends and family, but it was so much fun to have them all in the same room and to have my baby boy singing to his Mom, "You've got a friend in me." Having cancer gave me this gift.

The gift I did not appreciate was having no hair. I have never been fond of my appearance but take it in stride as being interesting. When the word "chemo" came up, I thought, "uh-oh." Luckily, Larry and all the men in his family are "follicly-challenged," so I was in good company. Of course, to fit me, I had to have a man's wig specially ordered. The first came in too dark, the second too white. Too bad. It slipped, I taped. It itched, I removed. I frightened small children and embarrassed senior citizens. I was called "sir" and I didn't care. One day, I left work late and alone. I figured no one would see me, so I plopped it on my head to walk to my car. Wouldn't you know, I met a security guard who was in a talkative mood. Once in the car, the rear view mirror had the last laugh, because I had plopped the wig on my head sideways! Moving right along to the wonderful world of scarves... I don't think I have seen that poor guy since that night.

Later, while in a coffee house in Boston, I noticed first one young bald guy, then another, enter the room. They were socializing with friends normally, and I wondered what stage of chemo they were in. Gradually, more young people came in until there were about ten bald guys in the room. I figured it was a support group out for an evening and silently wished them well. Then it occurred to me that shaving one's head is the style now! I was finally in the in-crowd! I also realized how immersed I had become in the world of cancer.

DESTINATION IN SIGHT:

Now that I'm finally a "survivor," I think my family, friends, and co-workers are the most grateful. I gave them all a run for their money. I have learned how much it means to have people thinking about me, hoping and praying. I will keep the greeting cards always because people took the time to think of me. I know that the flowers and gifts are expensive, and I love them all. When a decision looms, even a horoscope might help.

It is important to be able to work, to keep occupied, and to be able to relax and take care of myself. It is important to have insurance, to have enough money, and to share feelings and experiences with others who are in the same boat. It is vital to be able to sleep, to have questions answered, and to overcome depression. The support I received has been endless, but the real help came in moments, here and there, when I needed something or received something I didn't know I needed. I was fortunate to ride on the "breast cancer express" with so much support. Many types of illness are not as well funded or supported, and I hope those people have friends who care.

In looking back on the positive changes as a result of this ride, I realized:

- I am not invincible.
- I need to take care of myself, both physically and emotionally.
- I need to listen to my instincts.
- My family is closer now than ever, and my marriage is stronger and happier with each day.
- Everything I eat or drink matters.
- Everything I do matters.
- I am lucky that I was diagnosed when I was.
- I have a responsibility to all those who have seen me through this experience, to "pay it forward."

I will watch my ninety-three-year-old Mom and learn from her lifestyle so I can be there for my kids. It is only a disease; it is not my life. The important thing is to get back to the business of living! I will do that for me.

MY BIO

I consider myself to be a reasonable, deliberate, and useful person. I was raised in a healthy, happy family as the youngest of four siblings. Mom is active and healthy at 93. I am currently 59 years old and find wisdom for living from art, music, and the thoughts of others. I am an artist at heart and love to draw and paint anything, but especially elderly people. I was an art education major in college, but spent my whole career working in activities for long-term care. I retired in 2005 and work six different little jobs dealing with old people and old things. My husband and I have raised our two children in the same house in which his mother was raised. Larry is a substance abuse counselor, daughter Corey is an artist, and son Rob is a musician. My post treatment goal is to finish planting the garden I started two years ago.

$$\left(2\right)$$

Navigating an Uncertain Sea

BY PAT BATTAGLIA

*"I don't worry about the storms,
for I am learning to sail my own ship."
Louisa May Alcott*

MY DIAGNOSIS:

On May 7, 2004, I was diagnosed with ductal carcinoma in situ, or DCIS, a very early stage cancer that was scattered through approximately one-third of my left breast. In the midst of that was a more advanced lesion—an area of invasive ductal carcinoma, or IDC. Six weeks later I had a mastectomy, and the pathology reported the 1.4 cm tumor to be Stage I, nuclear grade 2. A subsequent lymph node dissection revealed that the cancer had spread to one of the eighteen nodes that were removed, and my condition was then considered to be a Stage II cancer. I had eight rounds of chemotherapy over a period of four months, followed by five years of hormonal therapy: two and a half years of Tamoxifen, then the same length of time on Aromasin. There is currently no sign of cancer in my body.

MY JOURNEY:

I've heard it said that the first thing you do when you hear you have cancer is cry. I didn't shed a tear when I learned of my diagnosis, and to this day, I can't say why. I remember sitting on the examining table in a darkened room, listening to the radiologist interpreting my mammogram as if she was speaking from a distance. Feeling as though there was nowhere to turn, I became detached, a member of the audience in a drama that was enfolding before me.

"I hope I'm wrong about this, but you probably have breast cancer," she said, and proceeded to point out details on the illuminated film that hung behind her.

My vocabulary grew as I listened. Scattered white dots that looked like a star map, almost beautiful, were "microcalcifications," the hallmark of an early in situ form of cancer. A larger white area among the stars that resembled a nebula was an area that could be "invasive."

My head swam, and a flash of memory flooded my consciousness. For a few brief seconds, I was carried back in time to the days when I had nursed my five children. A rush of memories overtook me in that short space of time, memories of the sweet smell and soft feel of a newborn, and the incredible feeling of nourishing a brand new life with my own body. Then a quick snap back to the moment—how could there be a cancer growing in my breast? How could this body, which had given life, also give rise to cancer? Finally, moving past the betrayal and confusion, I made a complete, almost instantaneous circuit through my emotions and came back to numb.

Until that point, I regarded the lump that had made its

presence known in the previous few weeks as something to be dealt with, a benign mass to be removed "just in case." My sisters had been down that road, and now I would join them. We'd share our stories the next time we got together. But at the moment the word "cancer" was uttered to me by a doctor, I knew I had taken a turn down a very different road, one I had never thought I would travel. I was full of apprehension about this unknown territory.

A needle biopsy followed shortly after the meeting with the radiologist, and my bewildered husband arrived at the office during the procedure. I had called him on a borrowed cell phone in the interim between meeting with the radiologist and the biopsy.

"What are you doing to her?" he asked the desk receptionist when he was told that he could not accompany me during the procedure and would have to bide his time in the waiting room. When I was able to join him, bruised and bound tightly around my breasts by the biggest ace bandage I'd ever seen, he hugged me carefully so as not to hurt me. His gentleness said more any great big bear hug could. We then joined the radiologist in a meeting room to go over the events of that afternoon.

My husband asked most of the questions as I sat feeling strangely detached and devastated at the same time. Questions were asked that could only be answered when the results of the biopsy were available: "What kind of cancer is this? What kind of treatment will I need? What kind of surgery will I need?" But other questions churned beneath the surface: "How could this happen to me? How do I tell my children?" And of course, the biggest one of all: "Will I survive?"

A short while later, at home with my children, I lamely attempted to explain what had happened and why I'd been gone for the whole afternoon. Feeling my way without a map to guide me, I launched into a description of how sometimes things go wrong with cells, and hadn't gotten very far when I was stopped cold in my tracks by a question from my thirteen-year-old son: "Do you have cancer?"

"Yes," was all I could say. I was grateful for his blunt perceptiveness, yet I felt exposed, the secret revealed. There was nowhere to hide. This was real.

That evening, I accompanied my son to his baseball practice and waited in the bleachers with other parents. It was the first practice of the season, and there were new faces to meet as I watched the team catching high fly balls and running plays. I tried to join in the conversation with those around me, feeling uncomfortably aware of the bandage that was still wrapped tightly around my chest. I felt apart from this group, an alien, even though I appreciated the distraction from the events of the afternoon.

"Hi, my name is Pat." (I have cancer.)

"Nice to meet you." (I have cancer.)

"Yes, this is my son's first year on this team." (I have cancer.)

"He's a good first baseman." (I have cancer.)

The events of that day stand clear in my memory, but my memories of the weeks and months that followed are a blur of doctor appointments and gut-wrenching decisions.

From the time I first learned that I was pregnant with my oldest child, through breast feeding and home schooling my young children, and on through several health challenges that my growing family faced, I gathered the resources I needed to make well-informed choices. Now, confronted by my breast cancer diagnosis, I felt compelled to understand what was going on in my body, so I began to read and research all I could find on the topic. I searched books, scanned the Internet, and quickly became overwhelmed by the scope of this thing called breast cancer. There are many factors and variables; it isn't a single disease. Each woman's diagnosis is as unique as a fingerprint. There is much information available—some excellent, some frightening, and some downright misleading. I was at a loss as to how I would fit this plethora of information into my own experience.

Through these early post-diagnosis days, I continued to feel disconnected, a solitary figure on a broken path. I woke from fitful sleep each morning, wondering if the whole thing had been a bad dream, and felt my breast to see if it was true. With each new day, I came once more upon the realization that this was really happening; the lump was still there.

One of the hardest things I have ever done in my life was to tell my mother I had breast cancer. A kind, sensitive soul, she was frail in body but strong in spirit. I knew she would want to travel the 2,500 miles to be by my side and help in any way she could. Her health made such a trip unthinkable, and as a mother myself, it broke my heart to think about how she would worry. But I believe in the power of a mother's love and knew that in her devout faith, she would pray as only a mother can pray for her child. I truly needed those prayers, so the words spilled out over the telephone, "Mom, I have breast cancer." She offered words of encouragement, and I promised to fill her in on every detail of my treatment.

A few days later, a card arrived in the mail addressed to me in her distinctive, swirling handwriting. The front of the card said, "At times like this, there's an old saying I rely on to get me through." The inside of the card contained this pearl of wisdom: "@#&%#&@!!!!!!!" When all else fails, verbal blasphemy to the rescue! I confess to resorting to this on many occasions during my diagnosis and treatment, and I have no regrets. Cancer isn't nice. It doesn't play by the rules, and I see no reason to always speak politely when dealing with it.

Four of my children were delivered by a midwife, and she continued to oversee my health care after my years of childbearing were behind me. She was the one to send me for the fateful mammogram when she felt the lump I had discovered in my breast. During the week after my diagnosis, she stepped in once again and set me on a course toward healing. She knew someone, a former midwifery student, who had gone on to direct an organization dedicated to breast cancer. I jumped at the chance for a human connection; I didn't know anyone personally who had ever been through this. When I called, the voice on the other end of the line was warm and caring, someone who had faced the same questions that were swirling through my mind. This person had somehow made it through, and now, on the other side of the experience, extended her hand to me to help me along my way.

The office of this local, grass roots organization is the site of a weekly lunchtime gathering of breast cancer survivors, and I was invited to join them. Sitting down at a table of women who were, or had once been, on a path similar to my own was an indescribably powerful experience. They talked and I listened. I talked and they listened. I witnessed firsthand accounts of women as they made their way through their own breast cancer experiences. I learned things that no book or internet article could teach about navigating excruciatingly difficult decisions and their aftermath.

Here were women facing life-altering questions and decisions: choosing between mastectomy and lumpectomy; wondering why chemo and radiation are in the treatment plan for some and not others; asking when to seek a second opinion; needing to know how to understand a pathology report. Amid the tears and hard questions, there were smiles and laughter. Healing laughter. I walked into that room alone, and walked out knowing I was part of a sisterhood. In the course of an hour, my sense of isolation was dispelled.

With the support and encouragement of the women in my local survivors network, I began to sift through the glut of information I had gathered and, bit by bit, pieced together my treatment plan. It became apparent from the extent of the affected area that a modified radical mastectomy was my best surgical choice, and that took place six weeks after my diagnosis. All the tissue was removed from my breast, but most of the muscle and much of the skin was spared. A small, temporary implant was put in place that would slowly be expanded over the next few months with saline injections. Eventually, in a separate procedure, the tissue expander would be removed and replaced with a permanent implant.

Nine days after my mastectomy, still in some pain, I sat in a local theater and watched with pride as my eighteen-year-old daughter graduated from high school. It was good to be able to participate in this rite of passage, to see my daughter bask in the glow of her special day. My discomfort paled in comparison.

My next step was to consult with an oncologist, who surprised me by recommending chemotherapy. I was uncertain of that at first, but then the cancer was found to have spread to one of my lymph nodes, and the whole picture changed. Chemo became part of my treatment plan. It left me bald, nauseated, and exhausted.

I relied heavily on the support of my survivor-sisters to lift my spirits during these days. My two daughters, the eldest of my five children, took over the care of their younger brothers when I went for treatments and on the days when I was too tired to function. When a friend who was working toward her license in Reiki therapy offered her services to me, I jumped at the chance. I found Reiki to be a gentle, restorative therapy that left me feeling relaxed, cared for, and ready to face the next treatment. Eight rounds of chemo, spaced at two-week intervals, brought me through the winter holiday season and into the new year.

My cancer was estrogen/progesterone receptor positive: it used some of the naturally occurring hormones in my body as a means to grow. So when chemo ended, it was followed by five years of hormonal therapy. That consisted of one pill taken daily, a drug designed to negate the effects of estrogen. Its effects were far reaching, and between the chemo and hormonal treatment, I arrived at a sudden menopause.

Two months ago, I completed the hormonal therapy. I am now fully out of treatment. Today I am a survivor by anyone's standard, but by my own personal standard, I have been a survivor since that day in the radiologist's examination room. The word "survivor" is much bandied about, but I feel that it applies to many besides those who have faced cancer. I've come to view a survivor as someone who is fully at the helm of the ship, even while navigating a sea of doubt. My own ship may be a small dot on the surface of a stormy ocean, but I'm in charge of that ship. I did not choose to have cancer, but I am in complete control of how I will face it.

A good measure of grief has come with this experience. There is a loss of innocence, of the feeling that breast cancer is a terrible thing that happens to other people. There is the loss of my breast. There is a loss of precious time in my children's lives that I can never get back, time I had to devote to my own healing so that we could go on as a family.

But there is not just loss. I have a stronger sense of my place in this world. I am a wife, mother, daughter, sister, and friend. I am a voyager in this world, one among many. I come from a line of women who possess a deep inner strength, and I am proud to carry that heritage. I am a pacifist by nature and an artist by temperament. Having faced my mortality, I have delved into my soul through prayer and meditation, and have discovered a strength of spirit in myself that I was only marginally aware of before. I am learning to let that spirit shine in this one glorious life that is mine to live. I lost a part of my body, but my true self remains intact and continues to grow, to learn, and to love.

MY BIO

In my life I have been an artist, a craftswoman, a retail worker, a doctor's office receptionist, and a self-employed seamstress. When my first daughter was born, I became a stay-at-home Mom. I earned the money to feed our growing family by doing family day care as my husband worked long hours building his own business, a retail store. Eventually the store grew to a level that could comfortably support our family, and I continued to care for our five children, home schooling most of them during the early years of their education. I learned to take a proactive stance in dealing with educational issues and various health crises that arose during this time. When I discovered I had breast cancer, this background served me well in dealing with my diagnosis and treatment. Since then, I have turned to writing and journaling to help me process all that has happened, an endeavor I had neglected since my college days. I have become involved with my local breast cancer group, and am now a staff member of that organization. My breast cancer experience was truly an awakening. I wish I could have come upon this in an easier way, but I gratefully accept all the good that life has to offer.

3

The Climb

BY MARGARET SCHULER

"There's always gonna be another mountain, I'm always gonna want to make it move, always gonna be an uphill battle, sometimes I'm gonna have to lose. Ain't about how fast I get there. Ain't about what's waiting on the other side. It's the climb."
Miley Cyrus

MY DIAGNOSIS:

I was diagnosed with breast cancer on September 20, 2006. My final diagnosis was intraductal carcinoma, hormone receptor positive, HER2 negative, Stage I. The 1.4 cm lump in my left breast was found during a self-exam. I chose to have a bilateral mastectomy and sentinel lymph node dissection with reconstructive surgery. I received four doses of chemotherapy (Cytoxan and Adriamycin). I did not need radiation since the margins were clear and there was no cancer in any of my lymph nodes. After chemo, I began taking Tamoxifen daily. In 2007, I had genetic testing done which showed that I have the mutation to the BRCA2 gene. After having a recommended full hysterectomy in 2008, I stopped the Tamoxifen and began taking Arimidex daily, which I continue to take.

MY JOURNEY:

It was August 2006, and my mother had me over for lunch to celebrate my fortieth birthday. I glanced through a published calendar depicting breast cancer survivors that she had on her kitchen counter. She said she had already read it, so I should take it home and read it as well. It told the stories of brave women who were diagnosed with breast cancer. Days later, I did a self-exam and found a lump in my left breast. I was shocked and afraid, but knew it couldn't be ignored. The coincidence was surreal to me. Later, I told my mom that she was my guardian angel.

After finding the lump but before being diagnosed, I read everything I could find about lumps and breasts. I kept checking to see if the lump was gone or changed. I read scary statistics on the Internet. I hoped for the best, but imagined the worst. I told no one.

The day my kids went back to school, I called my doctor and made an appointment. I then called my husband and told him about my lump and my fears. I couldn't put it off any longer. My husband's father had passed away from cancer in 1991. Talking about cancer made it so real.

I had a mammogram days later. It did not show the lump, but it was seen during an ultrasound. I had a needle biopsy done immediately. My sister waited in the waiting room for hours that seemed like eternity.

On September 20, 2006, the doctor called me at home at five pm. I sat on my bathroom floor with the door locked and a pen and paper in hand as the doctor told me that I had breast cancer and needed to find a surgeon. My emotional roller coaster began.

My husband and I hugged and cried as we tried to absorb this information. Telling our two young children, our families, and our friends was our first step.

My daughter (age 11) and my son (age eight) were sitting in my family room with my husband and me watching *America's Funniest Home Videos*. I find it strange that I remembered, since I usually can't remember what I had for lunch yesterday. We turned the TV off and said we had some news. I told them I had found a lump, and my hand immediately went to my breast. My daughter looked at me terrified. She knew what cancer was and that it was serious. She had read that calendar, too. My son wasn't sure what to think. I do remember him asking if we could call it something else, so he wouldn't have to say the word "breast."

I then began the task of telling our family and friends. Everyone was very supportive, which kept me positive. I had never felt more loved.

We then began the search for surgeons. I decided to have a bilateral mastectomy even though research and the surgeons I consulted with said a lumpectomy was an option for me. I knew I would worry if I wasn't as proactive as possible. I've always had very small breasts and thought, "Hey, I may as well get some new boobs out of this!"

My surgery was scheduled for October 13, 2006. Friday the thirteenth was going to be my LUCKY day! I couldn't wait to have the cancer removed. The surgery was successful. The margins around the removed tissue were clear of cancer, as were my lymph nodes. I was thrilled with my pathology report. My surgeon recommended that I meet with an oncologist to see if further treatment was necessary. I thought I was done, but also thought that her suggestion was a good idea.

Words cannot express how I felt when the oncologist gave me statistics for cancer returning if I did not have chemo and take a daily hormone drug. I thought the margins were clear, my lymph nodes were clear, and the cancer was gone. Why would I need chemo? Well, there was some microinvasion. Although the tumor was contained, the cell walls were permeated in two areas. It tried to escape and there were no guarantees. Life is like that.

I didn't cry during any of my doctor appointments until I found out that I would lose my hair. As crazy as that sounds since I was fighting for my life, that fact devastated me. I began chemo in November 2006. I woke up that morning staring into my closet, wondering what one wears to their chemo appointment. I chose a comfy outfit. My husband accompanied me there. My sister, parents, and mother-in-law sat with me as they put the chemo into my veins. They brought musical cards, stuffed animals, and most of all, love. Most of the other patients were much older than I was. They kept to themselves. Sometimes I felt like maybe having my family there was bothersome to them, but mostly I think it helped them pass the time. We weren't the quietest group, and we were trying to make the best of it.

My body accepted the chemo without too much difficulty. The chemo only made me a little nauseous, but the thought of putting it into my body made me emotionally ill. I felt like I was being poisoned, yet at the same time was grateful I was able to have chemo to keep me cancer-free.

After my first chemo treatment, I went home, crashed on the couch, and watched my family resume their normal activities. This made me happy. I was a stay-at-home mom and was the one who made sure family members were where they needed to be. I had to let others take over that role for a bit. At first I struggled with this, but then I knew I had to get better so I could resume this role as soon as possible.

Family and friends made meals, drove the kids around, and helped in so many ways. My husband was the best caretaker I could have asked for. I could not have recovered so well if it wasn't for him and all the people who loved me. I was overwhelmed by their generosity.

My sister went wig shopping with me. After trying many on, we found one we liked. I brought my husband back the next day to see what he thought, and $800 later, I walked out with a wig in a plastic bag. We went to lunch after to celebrate my purchase. The bag sat on the windowsill next to our table, "staring" at me.

I spent the next few weeks admiring everyone's hair while waiting to lose mine. As the days passed, I would tug on my hair. Eventually I decided to cut my long hair short. My close friend came to my house and gave me a GI Jane look. It wasn't too bad, just different. Then, a few days later, it happened. My hair was coming out in clumps. Since my hair was almost black against my white scalp, I felt like a Dalmatian. My husband shaved it for me as I stood in the shower and cried. He told me I was beautiful. I told him he was lying, but I appreciated it more than words can express.

I wore my wig religiously. I actually received compliments from strangers asking where I had my hair done. It did the job, and it was worth every penny. The only person who ever saw me bald was my husband. I sometimes wished I could be one of those women who walked around being proud of their bald head. Instead I felt like I looked like a cancer patient or an alien. I wore a hat around the house. One time, I leaned over and my hat fell off as my son walked into the room. My hair had just started growing back. We looked at each other open-mouthed until I quickly put it back on. I told him I was sorry. He told me I was still beautiful. Thank Heaven for little boys.

I survived the bilateral mastectomy October 2006, the chemo from November 2006 to January 2007, the reconstructive surgery in April 2007, and the hair loss. I received food, flowers, food, cards, and more food. I had genetic testing in April 2008 and found out I had tested positive for the mutation to the BRCA2 gene. This put me at a higher risk for many cancers, so I had a full hysterectomy in June 2008. There had also been an area of concern on my right ovary, but it turned out there was no cancer. In January 2010, I found another lump in my left breast. My surgeon removed it immediately and found it to be scar tissue.

I am a survivor.

Many people believe I am a strong woman. I never thought so, but maybe they are right. I know I want to watch my children marry, hold my grandchildren, and grow old with my husband. I've known this all along. My daughter once wrote a story about me being her hero. Thank Heaven for little girls. I want people to know that cancer can be beat. That early detection is the key. That being proactive is not a choice, but a necessity. Having a positive attitude is half the battle. I also know that there's always going to be another mountain, and I'm up for the climb.

MY BIO

I am a 43-year-old breast cancer survivor, but I am so much more. My family and I reside in Rochester, New York. I have a

Bachelor of Science in Education and taught third grade for eight years. Soon after my first child was born, I decided to stay home and care for her. My son was born a few years later, and I continued to stay home. I loved volunteering at their school and going on all the field trips. This past year, I began working part-time at my husband's company. It is interesting work with interesting people. I also enjoy gardening, reading, baking, and exercising.

My husband and I will be celebrating our nineteenth wedding anniversary this year. He is successful, handsome, generous, protective, and my soul mate. He enjoys golf, cars, hockey, and red wine. My children are busy with school, dance, soccer, hockey, and socializing with many friends. They are intelligent, beautiful, athletic, compassionate, and the light of my life. My family has been my ultimate support system. We enjoy vacationing together and participating in cancer fund-raisers. We are hoping for a cure soon. In the meantime, they are happy and healthy, and so am I.

4

Presents

BY JANE VALLELY

"God has given us two hands …
one for receiving and the other for giving."
Billy Graham

MY DIAGNOSIS:

April 1, 2005, during a routine mammogram and core biopsy, I was diagnosed with extensive intraductal carcinoma of the left breast, nuclear grade 3 with luminal necrosis and focal areas suspicious for microinvasion, and classified as Stage 0. My prognosis was excellent after I received 28 radiation treatments.

MY JOURNEY:

On March 28, 2005, I was up early getting my shower and hair fixed because I had an appointment that day. My husband was also getting ready for work and commented to me, "I thought you were not working today. Why you are getting all dolled up?"

Well, I knew exactly why, and I replied back, "I'm not working today; I am getting a Present."

He said, "Oh you must have a doctor's appointment."

He was right, of course; he knows me so well. You see, I have made it a practice to reward myself with a "Present" after I see a doctor or dentist for any treatment. I base this practice on being a Mom and remembering what I told my children when they were little and they had to go to the doctor: "If you are good, you might get a present."

Now that present might have been a new coloring book, a Matchbox® car, or even just an ice cream cone. At this age in my life, I could see no reason for changing this habit. I can now sport "Pap Smear shoes," "Mammogram Purses," and on a day when both procedures take place, that might mean a new outfit. I even have these "Presents" gift-wrapped and make a big deal when I open them in front of my husband.

Unbeknownst to me, this day would be like no other I had ever experienced.

After my mammogram and waiting about two hours for the results, I began to notice some women dismissed after arriving later than me. This gave me reason to feel that I was going to have to delay my "Present" shopping.

Sure enough, the sweet little clerk came out and got me, only to say, "The doctor thought she had seen a cyst and wanted to do a biopsy."

Now I have worked in a dental office for years, and I know the kind words the nurse says when there is something suspicious to be concerned about. I immediately called my hairdresser to rearrange my appointment. I had figured that a new hairdo, along with a new pair of spring shoes, would be my "Present" for that day.

After my wonderful doctor performed a core biopsy, I was sent home to wait for a call the next day with the results. Instead of going home, I did get the new hairdo. I figured I needed a little something, especially after the core biopsy (which really did not hurt).

On Friday, the caller reported incomplete results, so the lab needed another test. Now I would be lying if I said I did not already know in my gut what the results would be, but I now had to wait until Monday to know for sure. It had only been one year almost to the day since my last mammogram, and everything had always been fine in the past. Several years ago, I had a surgical biopsy performed, so I was thinking this could be a repeat of that procedure.

On April 1, 2005, I heard the dreaded words, "I am so sorry to tell you that you have breast cancer." No, this was not an April Fools prank; this was for real, and at that moment, I became someone I did not want to be. A statistic. Another victim claimed by breast cancer. A diagnosis such as this clouds your head with questions: How bad is it? What kind of treatment do I need? Who will do my treatment? What do I do next?

After hearing this news, my husband immediately became my "ROCK." He and I started a research program that clearly would have amazed any medical research team. We learned more information about breast cancer than we ever knew existed and more than we thought we would ever need to know. We also quickly learned that you cannot get through this without being completely informed of all types of breast cancer and what treatment options there are.

The next couple of weeks consisted of doctor's appointments, biopsies, MRI scans, and waiting for what seemed like an eternity for the results from all the testing. It was soon very evident that a mastectomy with reconstruction at the time of surgery would be my best choice for treatment. The possibility of postoperative treatment would be decided by a sentinel node test conducted during surgery, and it would determine whether the cancer had gone to my lymph nodes. A positive test result could mean I would need chemotherapy of some kind.

During the days leading up to the surgery, I received many phone calls, cards and letters of love and support, and a special blessing and anointing from my church. I learned how important it is to have such a caring family and so many good friends. With the support I received, I never felt like I would NOT be a survivor but did know it would take some time.

Many "Presents" I received after that trip to the doctor stand out in my mind, but one extra special one was sent by my twin brother. It arrived the Wednesday before my surgery. On the previous Sunday, he had gathered many of my family members and some close friends who happened to be in Birmingham, Alabama, that day. He had them all sign a bright red boxing glove to let me know I had all these people in the fight with me. That boxing glove gave me more hope and power than any of the people who signed it will ever know. To this day, I still have it neatly tucked away. Every now and then, I get it out and think what a lucky lady I am to have received such a meaningful "Present."

An additional gift that arrived from another brother and his wife was my "PINK RIBBON MASCOT." A mascot brings luck and laughs. Well, let me tell you, with its elephant bobble head and lovely, long-legged, ostrich-looking body sporting a pink and black net tutu skirt, this mascot brought me lots of luck and still brings me laughs. It also gave me the idea to look for items such as this and have them on hand to give to other newly-diagnosed ladies who would soon become my new friends. At a time like that, everyone needs a "Present." I tell them to enjoy this "Present" and if the need should arise, for her to pass it on with love, laughs, and a wish for good luck.

I had told my doctors that the one thing that was very important to me was to schedule my surgery so that I would be able to attend my son's graduation from the University of Chicago School of Law. When I look back now, I realize that his graduation was my focal point for recovery. I also know that I felt every bump in the road on the way to Chicago, but I made it and could not have been more proud of my son. For the doctors to rearrange their schedule so I could be at that graduation was a "Present" from them to me, and one I very gratefully received.

My surgery was scheduled to take place in May—on Friday the 13th. I figured I had already received the bad luck, so I was pretty safe having surgery that day. I felt very much at peace with all the decisions that I had made. On the day of the surgery, my husband and I held a prayer moment to ask for God's blessings and grace for each other and for my doctors.

I knew it would be a difficult day for my husband to wait for the surgery to be completed, so I secretly arranged for some friends to be there to support him during the six-hour wait. I did tell him some friends might drop by during the day to keep him company. He told me after we got home how much he appreciated me for thinking of that and how much he had needed their love and support during that day. Their gift of friendship meant a lot to us both at a time like that.

After four days in the hospital, I was sent home to rest and recover. I was completely overwhelmed by all the bouquets, meals, prayers, cards, and phone calls that came my way. These "Presents" were all such a lift and greatly appreciated.

My children—a beautiful, spirited daughter and a tall, handsome son—were living in Alabama and Chicago, and I had asked them to come after I got home, when I really felt they would be most needed. Their presence when I got home was such a "Present" to me. They quickly pitched in and helped wherever needed. My daughter made a great decaf mocha latté, since that was her part time job while she was in college.

When all the reports from the surgery were back, it was determined that I did not need any form of chemotherapy, but that six weeks of radiation would be necessary.

Today I am more than happy to report that I am cancer free and enjoying all the "Presents" God has given me. I've been blessed with family and friends, two wonderful sons-in-law, talented, caring, and selfless doctors, and a true community of love and support. But the best blessings are three of the most beautiful "Presents" one could ever have. They are my precious grandchildren: one beautiful little girl and two adorable little boys ages 2, 4, and 18 months.

Now after all the many doctor's appointments, mastectomy, reconstruction, and radiation, I could see something in my future other than shoes, purses, and outfits. I was thinking of something like gold jewelry, so as a surprise to me, my husband, the one who is still my "Rock," presented me with a gold awareness pin with a pink sapphire. I wear it today, but it does not remind me of the cancer and treatments. Instead, I am reminded of all the wonderful "Presents" I have in my life and how I can always pass on the spirit of loving and giving.

One thing I have learned is that "Presents" come in all kinds of wrappings. Family, children, grandchildren, friends, flowers, meals, cards, letters, phone calls, and loving acts of kindness like rearranging a schedule to drive someone to an appointment are all "Presents" we should not only give to others, but also receive graciously when they are given to us.

Breast cancer is something that is in my past, and I hope it will continue to stay that way. I am so thankful for the wonderful doctors, nurses, the medical community, and outstanding support groups that are still there for other women, if and when the day comes that they should ever need the same loving "Presents" of care I have received.

MY BIO

Jane Vallely is currently living in upstate New York with her husband, who has recently retired from a major corporation. After retiring from work as a dental assistant, she is enjoying her new career as a professional wedding planner. When she is not busy helping couples plan the wedding of their dreams, she enjoys time spent with her children, grandchildren, and other family members.

5

The Extra in Ordinary: Blessings from Breast Cancer

BY LINDA ALLEN

"The difference between ordinary and extraordinary is that little extra."
Jimmy Johnson, Football Coach

MY DIAGNOSIS:

I never felt a lump in my breast, but an initial screening mammogram showed it. Although I did not know it, my odyssey with breast cancer had begun. A second mammogram followed and then a breast ultrasound. A needle biopsy confirmed the diagnosis, and I was told I had infiltrating ductal carcinoma. I was in the office of my surgeon within a week of diagnosis and was told it appeared to be Stage I. The best-case scenario was deemed to be surgery followed by radiation therapy. In reality that was not the case. I underwent a left breast lumpectomy with axillary lymph node dissection. My estrogen positive and HER2 negative cancer was 1.9 cm and had spread to the lymph nodes in my armpit. I went home with a drain in my side.

I elected to be part of a research study to compare the effects of different treatments for breast cancer. I underwent twelve

41

biweekly chemotherapy infusions. The first six treatments were Adriamycin and Cytoxan; the last six were Taxol. Within two weeks of ending chemo, I started radiation therapy. All of this happened within the short span of eleven months.

MY JOURNEY:

I am an ordinary woman. I have the baggage of a woman embarking on her sixth decade. I have experienced some wonderfully high highs and been fortunate to have resources that have enabled me to do most of the things I have wanted to do. I have also been in the depths with some desperately low lows, wondering how I could muster the strength to get out of the messes. Mostly life has averaged out. I work hard and like to play. I am generally quite calm and in control, which is the way I like it. I wish my foresight was as good as my hindsight. I am the sunny person with a positive outlook and religious beliefs that give me strength and courage to get through tough situations. I have been divorced but am currently married. I have three children, (two married); two stepchildren, (one married); and five grandchildren. Lest I forget, I also have a beagle named Charlie. I think I am average, normal, ordinary; but for a period of time, I was out of my realm and definitely not in control.

It began with a mammogram. I usually have a screening mammogram done around my birthday, but one year I was busy caring for an aging mother who had fallen (at my son's wedding, no less). With her surgeries, rehab, and six weeks of living at my home, life went on around me and I simply forgot, so on my 57th birthday I scheduled a mammogram. It was done on Wednesday November 16, 2006.

I got the phone call the next day, on the day my granddaughter was born, that another mammogram needed to be done. I just knew in my gut that this was not a good sign. Suddenly life was moving at a pace I couldn't imagine or control. I couldn't research fast enough. I didn't want to know more, but I also needed to know all I could. Decisions needed to be made. I tried to act as if nothing was wrong, but something was very wrong.

Armed with as much information as I could digest and understand, I opted for a lumpectomy. The procedure was done in January 2007. When I awoke from surgery with a drain in my side, I knew the news was not what I was hoping for. I was not afraid. I just felt I had a job to do, and I was ready to get on with it.

Some days were good; some days were not. I healed from the surgery and my recovery was uneventful. I went to work as much as I could, and I marched on through chemotherapy and radiation therapy.

Throughout this whole process, there was a lot of "extra" coming before the ordinary. My life was touched by ordinary people doing what they were able to do with extraordinary grace and love.

My husband had lost his first wife to leukemia. He always reminded me that there was nothing we couldn't overcome, although I know he thought, "Why another time?" His strength is quiet, strong, and resilient. His love is just as quiet, strong, and resilient. In a word: Extraordinary.

My daughters expressed their love with a quiet calm that reassured me. My Marine Corps son, though far away physically, did the best he could to keep in touch with me. (They are special and extraordinary children, even if they are mine.) My wonderful stepson, who was in college and had no money but wanted me to know he was with me, sent me a pretty vase with daisies. He had learned first-hand what no kid should have to know as he watched his mother crumble from leukemia. I will remember his kindness always.

My girlfriend stayed with me on the night after my surgery when my family had left for home. We watched *The Letterman Show* together until I fell asleep. She seemed to know what I needed in that moment, and that night she put me before her husband and her beloved dogs. She gave me the quiet but extraordinary support of friendship and love.

Another wonderful friend got lost driving to my house on a windy, snowy, February night to bring a bottle of wine and to give me a pedicure and manicure. She had such a kind heart and gentle touch. I will never forget how she lifted my spirits. Extraordinary.

My college roommate called me every other Friday after a cycle of chemo to tell me her adventures as a respite volunteer with Alzheimer's patients. I eagerly anticipated those phone calls, which were so welcome. She was a breast cancer survivor who'd had a mastectomy six years before. She knew and she shared. She was funny and inspiring and extraordinary.

My eighty-three-year-old mom called me every day, just to say hi and let me know she was thinking of me. She took such good care of me as a kid, and I know she felt handicapped because she couldn't be in my home to cook the meals, clean the house, do the laundry, and just generally mother me. My brothers and sister sent lots of cards and books, keeping me in suspense every day, eager to see what would come in the mail. They made me look forward to every day.

My hairdresser of many years knew what was happening to me. When my hair was falling out in clumps, she worked me into a busy Saturday schedule, took me into a back room, and buzzed off what was little was left of my hair. Over and over she sent me cards and called. She was truly an angel. A couple times she did my makeup and gave me tips on what to do to "make" eyebrows. She was extraordinary then and continues to be an angel to me, even now. Her colleague, a male hairdresser who had survived cancer himself, helped me get a really good wig. He saw what I couldn't and got me the perfect style and color. He gave me confidence to know that no one would know that it wasn't my hair.

One Sunday I thought I had enough energy to go to church, only to find out I didn't. I fainted and made a huge scene. An EMT rescued me. He got me out into the fresh air and drove me home. I confessed that I was recovering from breast cancer surgery and the "hair" on my head was not my own. Was it on straight? He was capable, yet so very caring.

The priest called me at home that night to ask how I was. I know it's his job to care, but his words and gesture of concern and caring meant so much.

All these simple acts of caring and kindness made an enormous impact on my day-to-day walk through recovery. Extraordinary, life changing, every one.

Now I am three years post-surgery. I have residual side effects of neuropathy in my feet and hands from chemotherapy and I have lymph edema. I have scars. One breast is smaller than the other. These will always be with me. They will always be reminders, but it all seems inconsequential because I am… still.

My life has cycled back to ordinary. I work. I volunteer. I am active in my church. I read. I walk. I meditate. My life has returned to what is normal and ordinary. For a period of time when I needed it the most, my life was changed and enriched by ordinary people who took a few minutes to give me a little extra and, in my eyes, became extraordinary.

MY BIO

I was born and raised in rural Allegany County, New York, in the very small farming community of Cuba. With dreams of being a physical education teacher and coach, I graduated from SUNY Brockport. I went on to receive my Masters in Education from St Bonaventure University. Marriage took me to Burnsville, Minnesota. I raised three terrific kids and moved back to New York in the late nineties. I have taught school, worked for a plush toy company, been in the health insurance industry, retired, and currently work in a medical office in Canandaigua, New York. I live in the heart of the Finger Lakes with my husband Roger and our beagle, Charlie. I have three children, two stepchildren, and five grandchildren.

6

My Journey My Way

BY MARY ELLEN VOLLMER

"And in the end, it's not the years in your life that count. It's the life in your years."
Abraham Lincoln

MY DIAGNOSIS:

On April 30, 2009, I was diagnosed with estrogen positive invasive ductal carcinoma. I was 49 years old. I had two tumors in my right breast, which were found during an annual routine mammogram. One tumor was 2.2 cm and the other was 1.5 cm and was determined to be Stage IIA. I had a bilateral mastectomy with sentinel node biopsy, and five lymph nodes were removed. The lymph nodes were clear, showing no signs of cancer. My prognosis was good, and I had four rounds of chemotherapy. Reconstruction surgery was done in November 2009. I am on Tamoxifen for suppression of estrogen for five years.

MY JOURNEY:

Maintaining emotional balance and a positive outlook in the face of cancer's uncertainty was quite challenging. Looking back, I was in denial about the whole situation for a while. As I began telling friends and family, my strength encouraged them, as I said, "This is no big deal and I will get through this."

Some friends were quite emotional, but for the longest time

I never cried. I used my sense of humor to avoid really dealing with the news.

I said, "What a way to get a summer off and a boob job!"

The first time I really cried was when I told my daughter. She had come home for my graduation, but I did not share the news because she had to go back to school to finish her exams. I knew if I told her she may not have wanted to return to school.

About three weeks after my diagnosis, as we sat under my dogwood tree, I told my son I had breast cancer. I wanted to wait until my daughter was home from school; however, it became too difficult not to share with him. I found it incredibly scary to tell him I had cancer again after beating thyroid cancer in 1996.

He said, "Mom, you beat it the first time and you can beat it again."

We talked about what was to happen, and I said I really did not know all that would be occurring, but that I was going to have a bilateral mastectomy.

That week I drove seven hours to New Hampshire. During those many miles, I played over and over in my mind how to tell my daughter that I had breast cancer. I thought I would pick her up and take her to Strawberry Bank in Portsmouth, and we would walk the beach and talk. The minute I walked into her dorm, all composure left me. She took one look at me and wanted to know what was wrong.

We sat on the lumpy futon and we just looked into each other's eyes. I told her that I would be fine, but I had breast cancer. She looked like a deer in the headlights and said, "No, Mom, not you." She said that I had been through enough with my previous cancer and the divorce. We sat there and held each other and cried together. I had never cried so hard in my life, nor had my daughter.

She said, "I will be there for you every step of the way."

Little did I know my life would never be the same again, but she has proven true to her word.

I had a bilateral mastectomy on June 10, 2009. When I went in for surgery, I was cautiously optimistic because I did not know what they might find. I felt I had beaten it once, but could I dodge it again?

The day my daughter brought me home from the hospital after surgery, it was a beautiful spring morning. As we drove home, I recall smelling the cut grass and just appreciating everything I was seeing. It was like I was wearing different glasses.

I have experienced countless blessings going through cancer for the second time. As a single mom, I was always independent and found it difficult to ask for and accept help. Upon returning home after surgery, I quickly realized that I would need help. The support of my family, friends, and neighbors was immeasurable. I cannot begin to recount the numerous acts of kindness given to my children and me.

Parents may go a lifetime and never know what their children are made of, but I witnessed firsthand what an amazing young woman my daughter is. The day I told her I had breast cancer, she promised me she would be there for me every step of the way, and she did what she said she would do. She helped with the four drains, slept by my side for weeks after surgery, did grocery shopping and laundry, managed my medications, and drove me to all my doctor appointments.

My son was also a great source of support. He and I graduated from college within two weeks of each other. I am sure this was not the summer he expected after just graduating from college. Due to the incisions, I could not lie down to go to sleep for the longest time. A friend bought me a chair that reclined, which became my bed for weeks. Each night my son would carry the lawn chair up to my room so I could sleep in it. Each morning he would carry it back down to the sun porch, my recovery room by day.

Friends brought food. My son would come home from work and ask what had been dropped off that day. Both kids said we were eating better than when I was cooking!

We walked around the block every night and spent time together. In the past nine years, the children and I had taken only one vacation. I saw more of them in the summer of 2009 than I had in years. It was a special blessing to be home with the two most important people in my life that summer.

Another blessing was the neighbor who lives behind me. One evening, as my daughter and I were having our nightly walk, he asked why I was walking so gingerly. I told him I had just had a bilateral mastectomy due to breast cancer. He asked if he could say a prayer over me. The sun was setting as the three of us stood on the sidewalk. I have often wished that his prayer could have been taped, for it was one of the most touching moments of my life. He put his hand on my head and began asking God to bless my children and me. He also prayed that God would work through the doctors who would be caring for me on this journey and that my daughter and I would be blessed as we walked and shared this time together. He prayed that the memory of cancer not be only one of loss and pain, but also of the many cherished moments shared with those close to me. We hugged and I began to cry. I thanked him for taking the time to pray over my daughter and me. I never looked at our walks around the block the same way, nor took them for granted. Whether filled with laughter, tears, or silence, I cherished every step we took.

I gained a devoted and trusted friend on this journey, a professor I had in college. When I told her I might have breast cancer, she offered to be with me when I heard the news. She stood by my side every step of the way. She has e-mailed me almost every day since I was diagnosed. She went to my oncology appointment the day I heard I had to begin chemotherapy.

Initially the doctors believed the bilateral mastectomy would probably be enough, but pathology indicated that chemotherapy was necessary. Hearing I needed chemo that day scared me more than the cancer itself. The whole idea of hair loss, chemicals, and nausea was daunting to say the least.

My friend has taught me to be a better listener and to be patient with myself. The most valuable lesson I learned was that I could say and feel what I wanted to. She showed me incredible respect. I admire her intelligence, self-respect, faith, and zest for life. She has had a tremendous impact on my life, and I feel blessed to have had our paths cross. She gave me strength when I was weak and comfort when I was weary.

Another blessing to me and to my family was a rekindled friendship from many years ago. My friend would bring me groceries and treats. One day I was so sick from chemo, I called her to get Sea Bands, because I heard they helped with nausea. The nausea from the last chemo was so relentless that I was willing to try anything. Unfortunately, they did not work, but we laugh today at the idea that those measly bands would stop me from feeling sick. Had I not had cancer, this friendship may never have been re-established. We have just moved on and appreciate each day we have together.

Recently a neighbor said she felt privileged to watch me endure my surgeries and chemotherapy treatments. She said she had never witnessed true physical and emotional suffering before. We had an agreement that I would open the front door in the morning so she would know I was up and moving around. Many days she would poke her head in and would just sit with me. She said her children also witnessed something they had never seen before. The day I shaved my head, the kids wanted to feel my head. They thought I looked pretty neat with my bald head! She thanked me for being so open and letting them experience this with me. During my chemo weeks, they would bring get-well cards and post them on my refrigerator. Her daughter would ask me if my cancer was gone, and I told her we were working on that. They would come over and let my miniature dachshund out for me on the days I could hardly walk. I would be sick for about six days after my treatments. I would be so sick I would forget how it was to feel healthy.

My journey through cancer made me recognize that I was practicing religion, not faith. I felt a closeness with God on this journey that I had never felt before. When I was stripped of my health so quickly and suffered through chemotherapy, I gained a deeper need for my faith. Recently I became a Eucharistic minister. I hope to one day be there for others during their time of need. I believe I have survived cancer twice for a reason and need to pay forward all that has been done for me.

A big part of surviving this journey was my sense of humor.

My daughter made sure I laughed every day. A few weeks out of surgery, I wanted to weed whack my yard. I went out in my pajamas and weed whacked. What a sight I must have been. My daughter took my picture and e-mailed my friends to show them how crazy I was. It did not take long to realize that this was not one of my brighter ideas. The weed whacking ended up whacking me! I suffered for two days after that. I had never been this sick before and was frustrated by not being able to do things myself.

I love to work in my gardens, so my cousin came over quite often and worked in them. We both share the love and appreciation of gardening. She did so much transplanting by the end of summer that I think the plants were running for cover. I enjoyed supervising her and watching my gardens flourish. I cherish all the time we were able to spend together. She was also a breast cancer survivor.

The most humbling experience I had was when my daughter's best friend from high school had a Pancake Breakfast to raise funds for me. She wanted to get me help so I could continue to pay my bills while I was out of work seeking treatment. The outpouring from the parish and friends was so moving and like nothing I had ever experienced before. They raised enough money for me to make the fall semester tuition payment for my daughter. I so greatly appreciated all this family did for my family. It was hard to accept this gift, but I saw how much they loved doing it for me. I heard myself described as heroic, courageous, and inspirational. I never felt worthy of such comments. I was just getting through a day at a time.

One unfortunate part of this journey happened when I was let go from a prominent real estate mortgage company in the town where I worked. I was not prepared for this, but I plan to make this a blessing in disguise. I believe something better is out there for me. Losing my job has become more stressful than actually going through cancer. I feel like all I have worked a lifetime for is going up in smoke.

As I reflect on my journey, as hard and trying as it was, I would not trade the experience for anything. I have grown emotionally and spiritually in ways that are immeasurable. The friendships I have gained have enriched my life. I have met some strong, courageous, and inspiring breast cancer survivors through the Breast Cancer Coalition of Rochester. I am now a part of a club I never wanted to be a part of, but it has been a privilege meeting and sharing time with all those who share my journey.

I look at life through different lenses now and will always remember and cherish the goodness that was shown to my family and me. The greatest gift I received was the time spent with others and the depth of conversations and memories shared. Cancer added richness to my life that I never would have known without the disease. Each morning I awake is a gift. Whether I have another day or thirty more years, I want to live each day making a difference in the world. There was no right or wrong way to endure this experience, but I did it my way the best I could. Having had cancer was not only about suffering, but gaining a purposeful life.

MY BIO

I was born and raised on a farm in West Henrietta, New York, one of three children. I married in 1982 and divorced in 2002. I had thyroid cancer in May 1996. I live in Brighton, New York, with my two children, now 22 and 21. A lifelong goal was to complete my Bachelors degree. I returned to school in 2005, and on May 8, 2009, I graduated from Roberts Wesleyan College with a Bachelor of Science in Organizational Management. I graduated nine days after hearing the disappointing news that I had breast cancer and thirty days before surgery. I did not know that the journey ahead would bring suffering and unimaginable blessings and new purpose in life.

7

A Journey of Faith, Love, and Hope

BY BONNIE THIES

"Take in as much joy as you can whenever and however you can. You may find it in unpredictable places and situations."
Morrie Schwartz

MY DIAGNOSIS:

My original diagnosis in February 2002 was invasive ductal breast cancer with a tumor about 2 cm in size. Cancer had not spread to my lymph nodes. Treatment was lumpectomy surgery, four treatments (three weeks apart) of chemotherapy, and 6½ weeks of radiation. In September 2003, cancer was found in my lymph nodes on the same side as my 2002 diagnosis. Treatment was surgery to remove the lymph nodes, four treatments (three weeks apart) of chemotherapy, and 5½ weeks of radiation.

MY JOURNEY:

It was the sensation of walking into a brick wall. The wall had mortar sealed by the world's finest mason; there were no holes or breathing spaces. I distinctly remember standing in front of our bedroom window trying to look out as I was telling my husband Bill that the lab report confirmed the radiologist's belief that I did have breast cancer. There was nothing out that window; it truly felt as though the window had somehow morphed into solid red bricks. Then I heard Bill say that maybe they had made a mistake. His voice woke me up to the precious fact that this was much more than just My Cancer. This was going to ripple through my world, my family, and my friends. Then the tears began from us both.

The day before, I had my annual mammogram, scheduled at my usual time of 7:30 am. This had been my standard scheduled time for years. It got me in and out early and on with my day. But this day was destined to be different. After something suspicious was found in my mammogram, I was escorted into another room and introduced to a radiologist whom I had not previously met. This very soft-spoken, kind, and gentle woman began with an ultrasound of the area of concern. After this, she suggested a core biopsy be done. Although I wasn't overly anxious at this point, it was very clear to me that those around me were concerned.

After the core biopsy was completed, someone walked me back so that I could get dressed and then walked me to a small conference room. Within a couple of minutes, the radiologist came in and immediately handed me a large brown envelope. I quickly realized that it contained my x-rays.

Her words still ring with me today. She simply said, "You'll need these for the surgeon."

She then went on to tell me that she would call me the next day with the lab confirmation, but she said that she felt certain that I did have breast cancer. As I walked out of the building around noon, my immediate thought was how efficient they were, because it took them only a little over four hours to complete their diagnosis. Later I would think back on this moment to laugh and reflect that maybe I should have had something more profound to ponder than the time management skills of my radiologist's office!

To this day, I don't know if I said this out loud, but as the radiologist was telling me that she felt certain that I had breast cancer, my mind's immediate reaction was that this was totally and completely preposterous. Just months before, Bill and I had spent almost ten days backpacking over the hills and tundra of Greenland. We had hiked with 45-pound packs every day up and down some pretty good slopes and maneuvered through the permafrost heaves known as tussocks. Sitting there with her was the most surreal moment I had experienced up to that point in my fifty years of living.

A dear friend has said to me many times that there are no coincidences. So, my first non-coincidence was the grateful and happy news that our first grandchild was born on the same day that I received the lab confirmation of my diagnosis. My daughter and her partner were very proud parents of a beautiful baby girl, Kate Michelle. Since my daughter's partner, Beth, had given birth to our little Miss Katie, we all thought that her parents should be the first to be there with them. Michelle and Beth lived many states away from both set of parents. Our plan had originally been to go down a couple of weeks after the baby was born. This, of course, would be changing.

But, first things first! The birth of Katie was so very important. We decided that we in no way wanted to tarnish this event with the news of my breast cancer. We immediately began calling our family and friends to pass on this beautiful message to all. And, yes, our hearts were a little sad, because we knew that we would be calling all of these people later in the week with news of my diagnosis. Everyone was ecstatically happy for our family with the blessed birth of Katie.

There was no question that our daughter, Michelle, would be the first person we would tell about the breast cancer diagnosis. Towards the end of the week, Beth and Katie were home from the hospital, and Beth's parents had arrived to help. The time had come to make this difficult call. Of course, we wished beyond belief that we didn't have to pass on this news, especially during such a glorious week, but, as we all know, life is made up of many peaks and valleys. The peaks that we have experienced help to keep us grounded as we drift downward through our valleys.

I decided right from the beginning that I would tell Michelle and Beth all that I knew at any given time. We would all be on the same page and there would be no surprises for anyone. Our first conversation was full of questions from her and fewer answers from me, but she knew that the lack of answers only meant that I simply didn't know many things at that point, and not that I was holding anything back from her.

Yes, it was a ripple effect. Once we told Michelle, we began to inform our family and friends. We could feel the love and the support all around us. The ripple would go out and come back to us more than tenfold in the form of love.

It was during the first week that my solid brick wall slowly began to see some crumbling. The bricks were still there, but their mortar was beginning to weaken. The first crack was when I went to my own doctor, and she greeted me with an enormous hug and sadness in her eyes from what she had learned upon reading my reports. She began by recommending a surgeon and explained that he would guide me from there to the next step in this journey. This was the beginning of regaining some of the control that I felt had been taken from me, but the wall's crumbling genuinely occurred through the love and caring shown to us in the form of prayers, cards, flowers, phone calls, visits, welcome food, and special conversations from so many loving people in our lives.

My proposed treatment plan was to have a lumpectomy, including a sentinel node biopsy (which would determine if my cancer had spread to my lymph nodes), chemotherapy, and radiation. While I was in the recovery room after my surgery, Bill stepped in right after the surgeon had left. I was able to give Bill the good news that the tears he saw in my eyes were happy tears. The surgeon had just told me that the cancer had not spread to my lymph nodes. Once again, we shared our tears.

The chemo treatments began less than two weeks after my surgery. My chemo nurse assured me with much authority that if I should experience nausea after receiving the drugs, the prescription she gave me would more than take care of any difficulties. Well, I quickly became a skeptic. My vomiting bouts were spaced about ten minutes apart, and they lasted over thirty hours.

Next, we had another one of those non-coincidences. Our 24th wedding anniversary was that weekend! At one point over weekend, Bill asked if I'd like to take a shower. He pointed out that maybe a shower would help to make me feel better. Having had those 24 years of wisdom, I knew that I shouldn't say out loud the first thing that came to me, which was: "Do I really look like someone who cares about how she smells right now?" So, I politely said I just didn't think I had the energy right then. Later that day, we shared a cold can of corn for our anniversary. This was my craving, and with his 24 years of marital wisdom, he was wise enough not to argue with his smelly wife.

There were some highs and lows throughout the treatments, but generally things went fairly smoothly. With so much caring and kindness all around me, it made me feel that I could get through anything. I could feel the strength and love of those walking beside me.

As life began to get back to normal after the treatments, I continued to gain back my strength and enjoyed life to its fullest. I could sense the change. The change was not only in me, but also in those close to me. It is the small things in life that are most important: the moments we spend with family and friends, the phone calls we make to each other, the quiet walks taken with special people, the notes to loved ones, and so many other inspired moments in each day. We knew it before, but now we vowed to live it.

As our 25th wedding anniversary drew close, we decided that the following year we would take a trip to Hawaii with our adventure outfitter friends. Well, another one of those valleys was put in front of us; we soon had to cancel this planned trip. About 18 months after my first diagnosis, we learned that the cancer had, in fact, spread to my lymph nodes. The brick wall didn't appear this time because I knew how I would travel through this phase and was absolutely certain that I would not be alone.

After surgery to remove the lymph nodes, chemo, and radiation treatments, life continued solid and strong. My health came back, and we began to enjoy our hiking and traveling once again.

It was because of all that I received from so many special people during my cancer diagnosis that I knew I'd be able to somehow survive what came next. Just about a year after my second cancer treatments were complete, my husband died suddenly in an accident while he was cutting down a tree on our property. I still do not have the proper words to describe how I felt or what I went through after this, but all those around me had somehow been prepared with all that they had done for both of us as we traveled through the two years of cancer. The power of the rallying around me could be heard throughout the world. No one missed a step. Once again, their love and support helped to carry me along until I had the strength to do it myself.

As I began to heal from this terrible tragedy, I found it so comforting to be back outside and hiking through our beautiful world. One day as I was perusing the brochure from our adventure outfitter, I noticed a letter. Our friend, Rick, was asking if anyone would be interested in helping people with cancer while enjoying outdoor adventures. This led to me joining a group of people who raised almost $200,000 for the American Cancer Society. Subsequently, we all climbed Mount Kilimanjaro, the highest mountain in Africa.

During the training and climb, I met an extraordinary person. We shared a very special love and passion for hiking, climbing, and simply enjoying the beauty of it all. And, as another non-coincidence, he also was a cancer survivor. Two years prior, he had been diagnosed with prostate cancer.

Almost four years after I lost my husband, Jim and I were married. Our marriage was witnessed by over 170 people. These were all of the amazing people in our lives, many of whom had seen me through some extremely difficult times. Some had climbed Kilimanjaro with us in an effort to help all of our sisters and brothers with cancer.

Life is not always what we have planned. I have sincerely learned how important it is for each of us to find our own joy in what we know is truly important. What is important and joyful in your life?

MY BIO

When I received my breast cancer diagnosis, I was fifty years old. I had an amazing husband, an accomplished and loving daughter who was just beginning her family with her partner, and a very fulfilling career as an electrical engineer. Hiking, camping, and canoeing were some of our favorite ways to enjoy life and God's marvelous and vast world. We had done some adventure traveling in such places as Alaska, Greenland, Ireland, and England, as well as enjoying our own hills, valleys, lakes, and streams. Certainly there were the normal challenges; but I was truly blessed to be enjoying a happy, faith-filled, and active life.

Section Two:
The Human Spirit

Life is not always smooth and easy. The challenges of life reveal what we are made of, and the vastness of our strength is made perfect through surrender to what is and overcoming the odds. The Human Spirit may feel fragile at times, but it has a strength that adversity cannot defeat. This section celebrates the indomitable Human Spirit.

"The moment somebody says to me, "This is very risky," is the moment it becomes attractive to me."

KATE CAPSHAW

"Keep your promises to yourself."

DAVID HAROLD FINK

"Courage doesn't always roar. Sometimes courage is the little voice at the end of the day that says, 'I'll try again tomorrow.'"

MARY ANNE RADMACHER

"Will shall be the sterner, heart the bolder, spirit the greater as our strength lessens."

BEORHTWOLD, NEAR THE END OF THE BATTLE OF MULDEN
IN AUGUST OF 991 A.D., TRANSLATED BY J.R.R.TOLKIEN

8

Turned Inside Out

BY JUDITH ANN BARONSKY

"There is vitality, a life force, an energy, a quickening that is translated through you into action, and because there is only one of you in all time, this expression is unique. And if you block it, it will never exist through any other medium and will be lost."
Martha Graham

MY DIAGNOSIS:

The results of my last mammogram were fine, and then almost five months later, I developed severe flu-like symptoms overnight that made me very sick. The next morning, my right breast was red, sore, and warm to the touch. I thought it was an infection and made an appointment with my primary physician. Upon exam, he felt a firm area, but assured me there was most likely nothing to worry about. He suggested I go for an ultrasound anyway ("just to be on the safe side"), due to my family history. The ultrasound confirmed a lump. A biopsy was performed, and cancer was confirmed, along with lymph node involvement. I was diagnosed with invasive breast cancer.

The pathology report after my double mastectomy showed a lot of cancer in my right breast (who needs an exact number?), no cancer on the left side (hold on to the good news), with many lymph nodes positive (again, why sweat the details?) at Stage IIIB.

Prior to surgery, I had Adriamycin and Cytoxan A/C chemo once every three weeks for three cycles, then after surgery, more chemo, weekly for twelve weeks. Reconstructive surgery followed, and radiation is still to come. I will be on estrogen-killing oral medication for five years—my cancer loves the stuff.

MY JOURNEY:

It was the morning following my breast reconstruction surgery. I was at home in bed, still feeling blissfully drowsy from the OxyContin that I had taken around 4 am. I opened my eyes to see my ten-year-old son standing in the entrance of my bedroom, peering at me. I had not seen him since the previous morning. Before I left for the hospital, I had kissed him goodbye and had watched him get on the school bus. I missed him. I missed all of my children.

I smiled and said, "Good morning, honey," and I recall thinking, "Oh, what a sweet boy—he must be worried about me and wants to make sure I am all right."

I sat up a little to show him that I was not in any discomfort. He recognized that I was awake and came closer to me. Raising his right arm, he held up a pair of formerly white sneakers, which were now brown and caked with dirt.

"Mom!" he exclaimed, without pausing, "Can you wash my sneakers—they're full of mud, and what's for breakfast?"

The drowsiness suddenly lifted, and with anger in my voice I quickly replied, "Get those sneakers away from my ivory carpet, and where is your father?" I could not believe what had just occurred.

Prior to my outpatient surgery (which could have been an inpatient procedure, had I not had a strong desire to be at home with my family), I had made detailed lists, days in advance. In the moment, I questioned my decision. In the hospital, I could have had breakfast on a tray and a TV remote in my hand. I had made lists in order to ensure that my recovery would go smoothly. I had made lists because I anticipated a couple of days of relief from my daily chores and motherly duties. I had envisioned myself recovering from surgery while watching Audrey Hepburn movies and enjoying meals in bed while casually breezing through magazines. I did not plan to do the laundry!

Then, like a slap to the back of my head, it hit me! I smiled and I felt my heart warm, filled with love. It was then that I realized how truly blessed I was. Here I was, and the worst was behind me. The chemo and surgeries were now merely memories—they were all done. I had fantasized about this moment some ten months ago when my diagnosis was still new.

Now I am looking forward to the familiar sounds of a blow dryer once again. Soon my hair will grow back. Most importantly, my husband and three children are here at home with me (they are somewhere in the house, anyway), and even though no one is making me breakfast, we are together. I do not believe that my son arrived at my door because he really cared that his sneakers were full of mud. What middle-school-age boy would? He wanted his mom. He wanted me back in action, and after I yelled at him, I could swear I saw him crack a little smile before he left my bedroom. To him, Mom was back! To him, it did not matter that I had just undergone outpatient surgery. It did not matter that I was bald, physically altered, or emotionally drained. It did not even matter that I was fighting cancer. I was Mom!

Like a superhero, I could do it all. My son's routine request for me to wash his muddy sneakers made me feel strong and powerful. To him, I was indestructible. It was then that I realized that my role as a mother had carried me through the past ten months. All right, nobody pampered me—and thank goodness for that, since it would have made me feel more like a cancer patient than the fighter I needed to be. These days, most of these days, I love feeling like a fighter.

I did not always have the fight of a fighter, especially in the beginning when I heard those words, "It's cancer." Those words took me down in one punch and kept me down for days. I was dazed and felt like an emotional wet rag. More than anything, it was difficult to hear those sobering words. I am not saying it is easy for anyone to hear that they have cancer, but the fact that I had heard my mother say those same words in the beginning of her fight with breast cancer made it all the harder for me.

My mother had informed me that she had cancer over the phone, and in her next breath, she told me not to worry, that she would be fine. I think she purposely kept me in the dark through most of her treatments and doctor visits because she realized the seriousness of her condition. It was her way of protecting me. My mother died when I was 28 and she was 48. Her diagnosis also came when she was around the age I am now, 41. That was about 14 years ago, before my children were born. I miss her as much today as I did then. I feel as though she was taken away from me too early, before I was ready, and I hated the enemy that took her. It was ugly and ruthless. Though it still doesn't make sense to me, I have always felt a hole in my life without her, and even though they never knew her, my children have missed her steadfast presence as well. Losing her left a long-lasting sadness in my heart. I felt cheated, and in my mind, cancer was the villain. It was an ugly, ruthless, unfair enemy. My enemy.

In the beginning, when I first received my diagnosis, I especially longed for my mother, craving someone to care for me as only a mother could. For me, breast cancer felt like a horrible monster, and I was terrified of it. It was there lurking in my closet, waiting. There had always been the possibility that it would someday emerge, and I had hoped and prayed that the door would remain shut. I did—or at least, I thought I did—everything right to keep that monster away. I had yearly mammograms, scheduled annual doctor visits, and performed breast self-exams. I breastfed my children and tried the best I could to live a healthy life. It is still so hard to wrap my mind around the fact that I have cancer, just as my mother did.

It is strange, but my cancer journey has healed some of my wounds that went unresolved following my mother's death. I can understand now what she went through, both emotionally and physically, and why she made some of the choices that she did. I understand why she pulled away from me after she learned her cancer had returned and metastasized. At the time, I thought she was trying to get me accustomed to life without her, but I know today that her heart was breaking, knowing that she was leaving me behind.

The one thing I remember most from those early days after hearing, "It's cancer," is that I could not look at my children without completely falling apart. The thought of not being able to take care of them was overwhelming. I am so glad those days are over and today, through the support of my husband and children, old friends, and new friends that I made because of the cancer, my attitude is strong and hopeful.

Today, I am training to participate in a 5K race on Mother's Day, and life is good. It had been about twenty years since I last ran. I used to love running and do not really know why I gave it up. I could probably say that life just got in the way and I became too busy. Well, life came to a complete stop with cancer. I am different today for it. My husband and children are different as well. Even the feel of my home is different. We definitely do not sweat the small stuff anymore, and we appreciate just being together. We love each other and we laugh a lot more.

I learned something from cancer that I could not have learned any other way. I learned that I became a survivor the day of my diagnosis. I learned that I can trudge through anything, no matter what obstacles stand in my way. I learned that I have a healer inside of me. I learned that my family is strong and very connected, and we can rely on each other for love, support, and understanding. Most importantly, I learned that as women—and as mothers, too—we all have strength and a bond that, when needed, will shine. Unbelievable!

MY BIO

Born and raised in north central New Jersey, Judith Ann Baronsky is a nurse, a part-time dance instructor, a wife, a mother, and a survivor. She lives a blessed life in upstate New York with her husband Henry and three children: Alexander, twelve; Ryan, ten; and Lara, five.

"The truth will set you free. But first, it will piss you off."

GLORIA STEINEM

"What lies behind us and what lies before us are tiny matters compared to what lies within us."

RALPH WALDO EMERSON

$$\bigcirc 9$$

Am I There Yet?

BY PAT BERNHARD

"In time of sickness the soul collects itself anew."
Latin Proverb

MY DIAGNOSIS:

Final pathology report, January 27, 1992, six days post-surgery: Left breast, modified radical mastectomy—extensive infiltrating ductal type carcinoma of the breast (5 cm greatest diameter) with extensive angiovascular and angiolymphatic invasion seen. The angioinvasion is multifocal and seen in sections from the breast skin and in the quadrants. The tumor is present at less than 1 mm from the inked margin. Metastatic infiltrating ductal carcinoma extensively involving 18 of 18 left axillary lymph nodes with extensive extranodal tumor identified. This tumor is nuclear grade 3.

MY JOURNEY:

My journey began about ten days before Christmas 1992. I'd just begun my holiday vacation. My husband and I planned to go to Charleston, South Carolina, to spend the holidays with family in the Low Country. It would be our first Christmas without our children. Our daughter had been away for the last 18 months teaching in Switzerland, and our son had just departed for his first job in New Mexico. I'd had my annual physical check-up the day before and all was well. I left work that day in a good mood, ready to enjoy the coming weeks. First, I'd get some needed exercise before another day went by. I did a workout on a ski machine.

Thirty minutes later when I got into the shower, I lowered my left arm and felt a sharp pain in the armpit. I couldn't imagine what it was, but with a little palpating I knew the lymph nodes were very swollen and quite sore. I was 49 years old, in decent physical shape, and hadn't ever had a pain like this. I went back to my internist the next day; when he asked why I hadn't told him two days ago, I replied that "it hadn't hurt then."

He felt the swollen nodes, said it could be several things, and advised me to wait a week or so to see if it disappeared. If it hadn't, an ultrasound would be in order. I asked if I might have an infection and whether antibiotics might clear it up. He was willing to try that route first. My character flaw is impatience with "waiting." I'm really a lousy "waiter."

When I got home, I called the imaging center where I'd had a clear mammogram in November and scheduled an ultrasound. (Remember, it was 1992, before the insurance companies required referrals or approvals to determine who you could ask to take care of you.) I went in the next day and when the pictures were interpreted, the doctor told me how sorry he was to be the one to tell me. But he never said the word, CANCER and I DIDN'T GET IT! Maybe it was just denial of gross proportions, but I truly did not understand that he'd just told me I had cancer. Looking back, I wonder that I didn't ask him straightaway. Instead, I went off to Charleston with my antibiotics in hand, hoping it would all go away.

We came home early, just after Christmas, because I just couldn't shake the bad feeling. (Perhaps I had understood at some level in my brain.) I talked again with my internist. He'd had the ultrasound report, and told me I needed to call my surgeon for an appointment. Surgeon? Who had a surgeon? How little I knew, but now I was "getting it" and was most definitely frightened. I took his recommendation, called the surgeon, and got an appointment for right after New Year's.

It was really quite anticlimactic. The surgeon couldn't feel any swollen nodes and said we should wait for a few weeks and watch it. Hope surfaced, but I replied that I was "uncomfortable with that option" and asked for a biopsy that day (my impatience again). It wasn't quite three hours later that he called me at work to say, "We had a few problem cells" and could I "come to the office right now?" He seemed very distressed, and my hopefulness of only hours before took a nosedive.

As my husband and I drove home that day, each lost in our own thoughts, I kept trying out the words in my mind. I have cancer, I have cancer, I have cancer. I couldn't say it aloud, though.

Life as it was BC (before cancer) went on hold while additional tests were done, and MD friends were consulted for recommendations, for second, third, and fourth opinions. A general surgeon, a plastic surgeon, and an oncologist had to be interviewed and chosen. I worked by day and spent hours playing computer solitaire by night, because as soon as I closed my eyes, my mind went into overdrive. Uncertainty and fear were with me, especially in the quiet dark.

The doctors were now in charge of my life and would be in charge for the rest of that year. According to the calendar, there were 16 days between the visit to the surgeon and my modified radical mastectomy and immediate autologous transplant reconstruction with abdominal muscle and belly fat. It seemed like 16 weeks. Availability of appointments, my "let's do this yesterday" attitude, and luck in getting immediate OR time, were all fortunate, since the cancer was a nasty one.

My way of coping with this was to exert control over the parts of my life that remained mine, although I didn't realize at the time what my motivation was.

After surgery and seven days in the hospital ICU, I took an additional three workdays off and then went back to work full-time. When my scalp started hurting and the first handful of hair came out, I went to a barber and had my head shaved. I continued to work full-time, do all of my own housework, and not relinquish one bit of control over my life that I could keep for myself. But don't misunderstand: I was in full agreement with my doctors, and I embraced the protocols that they'd designed for me. That, in a convoluted way, was also about keeping what control I could. Chemo was my best friend. No ice cap to try and keep my hair, thank you. I wanted the chemo to go everywhere and wipe out every little one of those cancer cells in my entire body. I felt good as I went through chemo treatment, continued to work throughout, and didn't have many side effects.

In spite of all the needles, memory phase-outs, hot flashes, sudden menopausal status, and fears of the future, this was not a terribly unhappy time. I found myself meeting monthly with a fantastic group of women in a breast cancer support group. The original group bonded so tightly that the eight of us began to get together for dinner once a month at each other's homes. Nothing was held back! We could discuss ANYTHING together. We had endless threads going about the things that the doctors didn't tell you, the things they did tell you that were wrong, and the things that you could've told them. We laughed really often and really hard. These ladies were, and are, the silver lining to that big, dark cloud that drifted over all of us. We cajoled, encouraged, teased, listened, and when necessary, mothered each other. We shared our interests with each other and invited each other into our lives. One women's partner was unable to cope and left her (he did return several years later and they married), another was struggling with a new relationship and her changed body, and one was so withdrawn that she rarely lifted her head to speak. The rest of us talked frankly about our husbands' reactions. I remember being pretty unhappy that mine would never let me have a serious talk about dying. He just kept telling me (or himself) that it was not going to happen. I tried to stay positive, upbeat, and strong in all senses of the word. I was still really into the control thing, big time. I pushed the limits in much the same way that I did regarding physical challenges.

When I finished chemo in August 1992, I didn't feel at all liberated; I felt like the safety net had been pulled out from under me. Now, I was on my own without my little friends Cytoxan, Adriamycin, and 5-Fluorouracil helping me along and keeping me safe from the beastie. I was allowed to recover for three weeks and then a bone marrow harvest was done. After that, I began radiation for an additional five weeks. That really sapped my energy in the last couple of weeks, and I was, for the first time, very tired. I'd started this part of my journey early in January 1992 and finished in October 1992. My new hair was about half an inch long, curly, and stylish, and I didn't have to worry anymore that my wig would melt when I opened the oven door. I also made an unconscious decision that I would live life more fully.

One of the women in my support group was a runner. I'd listened as she had spoken of running as her way of coping with cancer. It sounded so interesting and different to me that I joined her, and for the next five years we ran road races of 5 km, 10 km, and one relay marathon. We kept it up until my arthritic knees finally shouted "ENOUGH!" I felt like I'd lifted a barrier during that time; I was able to physically challenge myself again, and I looked for every opportunity to do just that.

We have a local organization that started as a summer camp for children in remission from cancer. In 1996, they began a program for women who had had breast cancer. I went to their first "Adventure Weekend." It included trust games, scaling a telephone pole, and navigating a tight wire line 40 feet in the air. (We were secured with harnesses.) My first time up, I thought my legs wouldn't make it, I shook so much. The feeling of going across that cable with nothing under me was overwhelming. We did the exercise several times that weekend and, for fun, got to ride a 100-foot zip line from the top down on our last climb. I did more and more with this group and tried things that I never thought I'd ever get a chance to experience. I tied flies, learned to fly fish, and paddled a dragon boat, but best of all, I got a chance to try my hand at rowing an 8+ sweeps shell. Now, five years later, I still row four to five times every week and compete at local and national regattas.

Lymphedema is one of the persistent side effects from surgery and radiation therapy that I've learned to live with. It's constant and often troublesome, but I haven't let it stop me from doing the things I love to do. I know it's there; it's a part of me and my new body and life after breast cancer. Armed with a very positive attitude, one perceives that sometimes disease can bring you full circle and leave you with something other than pain, debilitation, and sadness. The Friedrich Nietzsche quotation, "That which does not kill us makes us stronger," applies here. I think I'm lucky that I've recognized the wisdom of that. I've learned that risk is relative, challenge is good, and the end product is often beyond anything you ever thought you could make happen.

I've been scuba diving in the Coral Sea and off the Great Barrier Reef, I've rafted down the Colorado through the Grand Canyon for two weeks, and I've trekked through northern Outer Mongolia for a month without knowing the language. Learning to live fully is a gift that cancer has given me. I don't save adventure or life for "down the road" or "maybe next year" or "let's wait till we retire." None of us knows what the future brings, whether we've had a life-threatening illness or not, so why not squeeze everything life has to offer out of every single day without regrets!

The month after we returned from Mongolia, I had another mammogram that indicated a precancerous condition in the right breast. The radiologist wanted to check it in six months. I'm still that impatient "control nut," so I saw a surgeon immediately and made arrangements for a second mastectomy. When the surgeon wanted to do another autologous muscle transplant, this time using a muscle from my back, I said, "NO! It will hurt my rowing!" so I chose a saline implant instead.

The strange thing was that having the "worst" happen, the thing that I'd feared and dreaded all those years was a non-event when it finally happened. It was not the catastrophe that I'd imagined it would be. I wasn't happy about it, but I knew I could do this again by taking life a day at a time until I came out the other side. I still wonder what the future holds and whether I'll have a recurrence or a new cancer. Meanwhile, I'll get in the hot pink kayak that I just bought and continue to keep rushing forward enjoying every day that I have.

MY BIO

The first baby to be born in the MASH hospital at US Army Camp Blanding, Gainesville, Florida, Pat Bernard was raised in Pittsburgh, Pennsylvania. She graduated from Munhall High School, Munhall, Pennsylvania (1961), from Allegheny College with a BA in Political Science (1965), and from the University of Buffalo with an MLS (1976). Pat is employed as the Director of the Henrietta Public Library, Rochester, New York. She currently lives in Mendon, New York, with her husband, a professor at the University of Rochester Medical School. She is a board member and officer of the Genesee Valley Handspinning Guild, a board member of Naiades Women's Oncology Rowing Program, and a member of the Genesee Rowing Club. Her hobbies include skiing, scuba diving, bicycling, kayaking, and knitting. She is the proud mother of a daughter and a son, and "Grammy" to three wonderful boys and one darling girl.

Breathe and Just Keep Running

BY ANDREA CARUSO

"You can only come to the morning through the shadows."
J.K.K. Tolkien

MY DIAGNOSIS:

On April 4, 2004 I was diagnosed with Ductal Carcinoma In Situ, (DCIS), non-encapsulated (movement within the left breast), Stage IB. Lymph nodes were defined as not affected, though it was considered to be large and appeared "on the move."

June 10, 2004, I underwent a full mastectomy of the left breast and lymphectomy with reconstruction through the free flap procedure (Tummy tuck!—Hooray!), then four months of chemotherapy followed by six weeks of daily radiation treatments. To date, there has been no recurrence! Every day is a blessing.

MY JOURNEY:

The diagnosis and treatment of breast cancer can sure mess up some of the best-laid plans. My nursing assignment in New York City required an annual medical physical, including a mammogram. My plan was to get the medical clearance I needed and return to my new job in an insanely busy labor and delivery unit. It was spring, time to be outside enjoying the city and running in Central Park.

On that rainy spring day in 2004, after my mammogram, I was called back down the long hallway to my exam room to hear the news that would consume the next eight months of my life. I had breast cancer.

The words at the end of the mammogram, "Andrea, you have breast cancer and it must come out" turned this usually rational nurse into a delusional one. My response to the news was to attempt to schedule surgery, chemotherapy, and radiation around my job in New York. When rational thought returned to me through gentle guidance from the wise doctor, I made plans for a mastectomy and reconstructive surgery, chemotherapy, and radiation that took place from June until December of 2004.

Spring and summer are busy times in the Northeast as the melting snow draws everyone outside again for sun, barbeques, and yard work. These two seasons are particularly busy for me, as I take an already-overfilled plate as a single mom and night nurse and add training for the New York City Marathon. The marathon was another concrete thing in my world that just didn't have time in its schedule for cancer. Due to my flimsy training habit of running nary one foot during my winter hiatus, it was always crucial for me to hit the pavement as soon as the snow melted. As fixed as I was on accomplishing this race every year, I had no idea the 26.2-mile trek of pure masochism would morph into a divining rod, leading me to streams of hope and strength that seemed to pour in and over me. I have always had a firm confidence in the source of my spiritual strength and hope, but this race, that year, was divinely placed as a finish line to aim for, representing distance run in miles and in treatment.

Preparing for a marathon often can bring guilt from inadequate training, feet that even daily pedicures couldn't make appealing, and shoe expenses that rival the national debt. I whine so often during the training phase of the marathon that more than a handful of friends have asked why I keep doing it. That question has now been answered for me beyond any doubt. I have learned repeatedly that things in life find their value in our hearts and minds as soon as something threatens to take them away.

My doctors pleaded with me to skip the race during that year of surgery and intense treatment. However, I became more driven because of, and possibly in spite of, the pleas not to run. After thirty years of running, the race took on a role in my world that it never had before. Working in a hospital during immunity-zapping chemotherapy was not an option; therefore, running became my new job. It became therapy, an escape. Surprisingly important was the statement of triumph it allowed me to make with every sweaty step. It screamed into my numb, fear-saturated ears that I was okay, that I would continue to be okay. After all, how sick could I be if I just pulled off a ten-mile run? My medical mind knew that my body could have been spreading the cancer, even as I ran, but my heart and emotional mind needed to feed on the hope that as I conquered the challenge of long miles, I was also conquering the uninvited invader in my body.

Surgery itself isn't an unknown entity to me. I have had experience being on both sides of the table. I knew the surgery ahead of me would involve many areas of my body and require a lengthy recovery. I had many appointments with my mirror as I looked at my breasts, the one invaded, the one not. Why was one attacked and the other passed over? Would they still be familiar to me even after cutting-edge reconstruction? I even spent a few mournful moments saying goodbye to the "sick" one, mentally thanking it for feeding my babies and being a part of my body for 45 years. I giggle in retrospect at myself for doing this and think that there is a psychologist out there who could have made a lot of money off me.

As silly as my actions seemed, I was comforted by giving myself carte blanche permission to feel anything I wanted to, express anything I needed to, or to not react at all if a shutdown phase came blowing through. At times, this permission rule allowed me to go a bit too far, especially if any pain medications had been ingested. The day I was to leave the hospital, I found out I would be leaving with two cumbersome drain bulbs dangling down from my abdomen. I gave myself permission to ask the sweet and unsuspecting resident examining me for discharge how he or any guy could tolerate walking around all day with two things dangling between their legs. He, being more gracious than I, chose not to respond.

Days passed, busy with post-op appointments and chemotherapy infusions, usually followed by admission into my "Chemo Witness Protection Program." I would go undercover, waiting for the haze to pass, gauged by how soon I was ready to eat food because I wanted to, not because I had to. Wanting to eat usually also meant I was ready to engage with humans again, to return calls, to drive myself to my youngest daughter's lacrosse games, even if I just stayed in the car and watched her from afar.

Though every chemo treatment was followed by days of plummeting layers of nausea, fatigue, and dizziness, I naively thought each day, "There, this is as low as I can go; this has to be the bottom; I will surely feel better tomorrow." Tomorrow always showed up, bringing joy in things that brought joy before: the sun streaming through sheer curtains, my precious golden retriever looking on with hopeful eyes that I might actually pet her with vigor that day. The fog always lifted, my make-up and wig went on, running sounded good again, and the horizon of one more treatment was in the rearview mirror.

These are the days, the connected moments that cause us to unearth the greatest discovery: what we are truly made of. This discovery is not fashioned with bricks of what impresses others, gives one a great credit score, or lands one on a magazine cover. These bricks are made with mortar found only in perseverance, the core drive not to succumb to the will of the cancer and its subtle whispers to give in and give up.

Ironically, some of these bricks are made of acceptance and gratitude at a time when being grateful seems at odds with what is happening. A dear friend gently suggested that psychotherapy might be in order, as she felt I seemed a little too contented. She was concerned that I was in denial and might hit a brick wall when the reality of my situation set in. It was then that I discovered the difference between denial and the brick called faith.

Every new brick I discovered renewed me. Bricks tell us to run marathons with no hair; they loudly whisper to stop and smell everything, not just the roses. They are bricks that build us up, yet seem only to come to us through challenge and hard work, even threatening our lives, with the outcome of a stubborn internal profession never to give up.

Every ballplayer who has lost by a half-court throw at the buzzer or a field goal in overtime can go home on the bus remorseless, knowing all was given, individually and as a team. We all thrive and survive best when we have a strong team on the field around us. I had that team.

The strong defenders on my team included my doctors who, with tireless brilliance and compassion, gave me the confidence to fight. They brought me to tears when they accepted that I was going to run the marathon anyway and adjusted my treatments to allow for it. I had friends and family who held my feet to the fire with their questions: "How are you? What can I bring you? Will you call me when it's bad, not just when it's good?" My daughters poured love out in their eyes, trying to mask their tears of fear. I suspect they also looked the other way when chemo brain would cause me to forget what I had said or a name I should surely have known.

My mother, my strong mother who has endured much and is given to sarcastic humor as much as avid affection, shrouded me with maternal love. She knew I was gingerly washing and brushing my hair as my head tingled and more hairs showed up on my pillows and sweaters. My mom knew that losing my hair would be one of the hardest hoops for me to get through, especially alone. She, after all, witnessed my development into the girlie-girl I am today.

Mom joked, "Look, your brothers have gone bald; I want to be here when one of my daughters does. Besides, I want to see you in your wig; it's just like your hair, only better!"

Her jokes got me into the bathroom for another session with the mirror. This time it wasn't to bid farewell to my breast, it was to brush and brush until almost every hair was gone. In twenty minutes, I transitioned from a forty-five-year-old woman into an eighty-year-old man.

My mom was waiting in the living room and greeted me with another joke, "See, I always said you had a good head." She hugged me, fought back tears, then helped me adjust my new best friend, my wig.

Just before leaving for the airport the next day, my joking, loving mother held my bald head on her lap, stroking where there once was hair, and professed in a cracked voice, "If I could take this into my body and do it for you, I would; I would."

These are the gifts that come from enduring much. I received the gift that hopefully none of my siblings will have to receive. I got to re-experience my mom as the mother of a toddler, who kissed boo-boos and made everything all better. She couldn't make this all better, but the message of love enveloped in so much "wanting to" was my gift that day.

My team, my all-star team, was quarterbacked by my only sister, who immediately upon hearing the news sent cards reminding me to breathe, to hang in there, telling me she was with me through this. Her sense of helplessness at being 3,000 miles away burst through her voice and words as she valiantly tried to control the uncontrollable. She had a vendetta to settle as well. When I had just heard the news myself, I called from the clinic, knowing our 3-hour time difference meant I would just be catching her at work. All I got out was, "Hey, they just told me I have breast cancer; oh, the doctor is back I have to go." I wasn't able to call her for four hours, something she should be forgiving me for any day now.

My sister stepped into her high gear sister mode and was set on conquering it with me. The tears passed and planning took over. Her very effective form of love is to control and fix all that she can and hold hands and pray for what she can't. Once she arrived, she made sure everything was managed from pillows, linens, and lamps, to a bedroom and a refrigerator stocked to capacity. She was the last face I saw before going into surgery, and she was waiting with thumbs up when anesthesia wore off. Holding her thumbs high up was the quickest way for her to let me know the surgeon stopped by to say that no lymph nodes appeared involved. My sister was my maid, my accountant, my chaperone, my prayer warrior, and the one with whom I could safely break down.

I tried to protect my mother from the pain of not being able to help her child. I shielded my daughters from seeing a fearful mother, knowing that if they saw fear in me, then they would be anxious about things they could not control. My shield could come down with my sister, whose care and concern didn't leave when she boarded the plane. She knew I was headed for financial struggle as treatment continued and my income steadily dropped. She sent checks for my mortgage attached to messages conveying that if I tore them up, she would have to fly 3,000 miles to do the same to me. It was humbling to accept the help, but it was critical in allowing me to focus on getting better.

My team aided my trek back to health, much like the graduated steps of training and running a marathon. There are strong and weak days, both in training and treatment, times of great strides and times of losing ground. I believe we are called to embrace both equally, trusting that we will be shown why in good time.

As a result of embracing it all, a shining gift was shown to me. With the hard work of a marathon and the example of generosity from my kind sister, I saw that other women in the same place of need that I was could be helped. The answer arrived before the question, "Why me?" I now knew why. I founded a non-profit organization to be the "sister" to those in need who, unfortunately, haven't been blessed with a sister like mine.

The organization that sprang forth from my sister's generosity is aptly named S.I.S. (Sustain Inspire Survive). Her simple and loving act of paying my mortgage for four months during my treatment became the impetus for the S.I.S. mission: to financially assist those struggling during the battle of breast cancer. Formed in late 2005, S.I.S. was the proud donor of nine grants of $500 each to patients that first year. By early 2010, over 400 patients have received grants, with over $250,000 being raised thus far. Funds are raised through events, grants, and donations, creatively involving businesses, healthcare systems, individuals, as well as patients and many generous volunteers. S.I.S. is a 501(c)(3) non-profit, United Way Designated (2440) organization. See www.helpSIS.org for more information.

The 2004 New York City Marathon records my slowest, yet proudest, finish time. I called my sister when I was done.

MY BIO

I am a single mother of two daughters, Lauren and Hannah, a labor and delivery nurse, a marathon runner, and a six-year breast cancer survivor. I am the founder of a non-profit organization (S.I.S.), created to financially assist those battling breast cancer. I have lived as many years growing up in Southern California as I have as an adult in New York, and have come to prefer snowstorms to earthquakes.

11

Breast Cancer Year 2006

BY ALISON CURRIE

"Life is the cookie."
Rachael Remin

MY DIAGNOSIS:

Right after Christmas, I consulted a surgeon for a hernia repair. Fortunately, he offered a breast exam as part of the overall evaluation. My seemingly normal lumps and bumps felt suspicious. Four days later he was proven correct. I was diagnosed with invasive ductile carcinoma with lobular features—breast cancer, at age 49. Happy New Year!

Thus began the wild, wacky, and not so wonderful Breast Cancer Year 2006. In a house with the motto, "Suck it up snot-boy!" I vowed to face my cancer head-on while maintaining my dignity, sanity, and sense of humor. What follows is a sampler of my emails to friends and family during this time.

MY JOURNEY:

MARCH 07, 2006

One down, seven to go. We had great facilities, free parking, kind, helpful, and professional nurses, and tulips in the window. Treatment took three-and-a-half hours, including filling prescriptions on the way home. My medi-port, a.k.a. the fiendish-thingy for you Beatles fans, worked well. One of the drugs was bright red, and its color made a second appearance later. Flush twice!

I experienced nausea only when explaining "quotients" to my daughter Maria. My family accused me of being spacey. I didn't agree, but maybe I just couldn't tell. We walked the dog this morning and I hope to jog tomorrow. I'm permitted to do what's normal if I promise to back off when necessary. John has threatened to chain me to the couch if I don't behave, so no Boston Marathon for me this year.

MARCH 11, 2006

Five days since my first chemo and I'm nearly human again. They detained me for thirty minutes after Wednesday's Neulasta shot in case of a bad reaction. Scary. Later, I fell asleep while eating lunch and awoke five hours later. I was wiped out the next day too, but finally felt better by Friday. My wig/"cranial prosthesis" search went well; the stylist made it fun, and I've learned that my head is non-standard and large. The post-wig-shopping lunch provided the first appealing food since Monday. Activities today included the world's slowest three-mile run, Maria's swim meet, and Andrea's All-County concert.

MARCH 14, 2006

In the words of Mark Knopfler, "*Sometimes you're the windshield, sometimes you're the bug.*" Saturday was a "windshield" day. "Life is Good," just like the t-shirt says. Then bang! Huge searing pains erupted on my right breast where a high-tech vacuum cleaner had hoovered out suspicious tissue for a biopsy. This was total agony, worse than anything I remember, and that's saying a lot.

We attended *The Lion King* Sunday night (suck it up, snot-boy), but I was in agony. Afterwards, I started running a fever and couldn't take it anymore. The cancer hotline recommended that I go to Emergency. No thanks! I contacted my (exalted) surgeon, who examined me and prescribed killer antibiotics for an infection. Our dog Bess could sympathize, as she was taking Cipro for a bladder infection. Misery loves company, but Bess loves everyone.

I survived Monday despite brief gut-wrenching pains after lunch; we have our own "big salad" story ala *Seinfeld*, bringing to mind the "don't eat the scallops" story, but I digress…

MARCH 16, 2006

It's getting strange. Food has become scary; spicy things are banished. I didn't understand the "chemo-brain" warnings. Now I do. I purchased a sectioned pillbox, because I can't remember if I've taken my medicines. Now, if no pills are left at the end of the day, I'm good! I should buy a blonde big-hair wig, drive a TransAm, and change my name to Debi with a star over the "i." I feel that ditsy.

There's always a caveat:

It would have been a great __(1)__ except for ___(2)___.

(1)	(2)
Pathology report	it was wrong
weekend	the infection
medi-port	what happened
sandwich	the chipotle sauce

When asked for advice for fellow cancer patients, Warren Zevon responded, *"Enjoy every sandwich."* I understand that: appreciating what you have, finding the good, and not sweating the small stuff. For us detailed, regimented, engineering types, it's not easy. I crave time with my family, rubbing the dog's belly, and doing the things I've "always" wanted to do. Enjoy every sandwich. Just make sure there's no chipotle sauce.

MARCH 18, 2006

"Out, damned port! Out, I say!" Not exactly *Macbeth*, but my medi-port started to swell and turn red. By Thursday, the pain was so unbearable that I couldn't shift into first gear. By Friday, the pain was searing. One look and my oncologist said, "That needs to come out. Now!" Off to the vascular surgeon's office where I sat, waiting, watching the redness grow, knowing they couldn't see me writhing in pain. Score! A surgeon came in hastily apologizing because he had someone "on the table." Three hours later, I was in recovery after emergency surgery. Killer antibiotics couldn't stop the infection, so my port had to go.

I was released the same day and felt infinitely better. No medi-port for me; I was just unlucky. I used something once that was good for 6,000 uses. It hardly seemed fair and delayed my second chemo treatment. John has been trained to care for my gaping chest wound twice a day until it heals. Lucky him. Always expect the unexpected.

MARCH 24, 2006

The call from the governor came through. I'm free! Today's offering from the *"You Might Be a Redneck If…"* calendar: "Your hospital uses jumper cables as a defibrillator." That's one service I didn't need.

After removal of my infected medi-port, oral antibiotics couldn't stop the infection. I remained feverish and the red area was spreading. The heinous port incident won me a 5-day all-inclusive vacation in the vascular surgery ward which, if you're sick, is the place boasting excellent nurses, technicians, physician's assistants, surgeons, oncologists, infectious disease specialists (wearing Prada shoes no less), and probably a partridge in a pear tree! Thursday was the worst, but things finally improved.

I blew four IV's during my stay and one before emergency surgery, ("You're not awake." "Yes, I am." "No you're not." "Yes I am." "We need a second IV here!" "Zzzzzz."), so the medi-port had been a good idea. I've met the all-star "IV" and "PICC" teams and proudly sport a peripherally inserted central catheter for future chemo treatments. Now running, weight lifting, vacuuming, and repetitive arm motions are prohibited. Walking remains okay.

As Dan Fogelberg would say, this was not "part of the plan." My hair began falling out in chunks on Thursday. My nurse told me I could buy great-looking head scarves like hers at the local Halal market. We agreed the ones featured in the ubiquitous cancer catalogues were hideous. Yesterday's *You Might Be a Redneck If...* offering was: "Your birthday cake is a pan of cornbread with a candle stuck in it." Today was John's birthday and with my breakfast came the world's largest corn muffin. Thus, I was able to provide a birthday cake (alas no candle) for my longsuffering husband. I'm hoping for a better weekend.

APRIL 09, 2006

"I saw a werewolf drinking a pina colada at Trader Vic's. His hair was perfect..."

WARREN ZEVON

Perfect hair days are mine, thanks to my cranial prosthesis. I've received countless compliments on my stylish, highlighted "haircut." At home, I assume a Syrian look, courtesy of my Halal market scarves. (I passed on the goat, but did purchase halvah.)

I've recovered sufficiently to resume chemotherapy on Monday. My gaping wound is steadily shrinking and no longer requires packing; Neosporin will do, so my home nurse/husband is grateful. Hi ho, hi ho, it's off to chemo I go! Let's get this over with!

APRIL 21, 2006

I was wiped out and slightly queasy after Chemo #2, but woke up rejuvenated on Saturday. While daughter Andrea toured Europe with the youth orchestra, we non-jetsetters drove to visit my sister on Cape Cod, where we beach combed, ate Easter candy, shopped, and flattened stuff on the railroad tracks. After my daughter and her cousin perfected coin flattening, they went on to the main event: Train vs. Marshmallow Peep. No contest. We watched the Boston Marathon and Red Sox game from a bar for the second year in a row. An injury kept me from running my second "Boston" in 2005. Next year, I hope to avoid the third annual "Marathon Bar Watch" and run instead!

MAY 03, 2006

Chem #3 went fine, delayed with the ongoing Chemo-Cribbage tournament tied 1 to 1. Once again, I was tired until Saturday's rejuvenation. Baggy sweatshirt season is ending, temperatures are rising, and t-shirt season is approaching, so off to the discreet (and pink) breast prosthetic shop on Park Avenue to fill the post-mastectomy void. The saleswoman was very professional with a wacky sense of humor and, after some comical misfits, I was able to purchase a balanced look. If only my new parts were bionic and could make me a Six-Million-Dollar Woman (anyone remember Lindsay Wagner?), but the only bionic result will be super slow-mo running.

College update! Andrea has chosen Williams College; rumor has it that kids are turning down Harvard for Williams. It's a great school, and nothing beats the Berkshires. Sadly, a wonderful woman died unexpectedly on Thursday leaving a son in Andrea's class and a daughter two years older. What a reminder that I'm lucky to be alive and able to fight this disease.

Enjoy every sandwich.

MAY 20, 2006

Like Huey Lewis and the News, *"I've Got a New Drug."* Having survived round #4, it's on to Part II: four doses of Taxol at two-week intervals. For the first treatment, I'll be at the hospital in case I react, turn red, or blow up like a balloon. I'm very apprehensive, but hope to return to my plush non-hospital setting for the final three treatments.

In addition to playing horn for *Pirates of Penzance*, there have been multiple concerts, recitals, and rehearsals to attend. My daughters and I ran the Breast Cancer Coalition of Rochester Mother's Day 5K run. Because of my PICC line, I hadn't run since March, so it was magic to run despite my slow-moving one-armed style. Next year, I'm shooting for a placement award in the "survivor" category. Today is my fiftieth birthday, and I'm happy to have made it this far.

MAY 23, 2006

Taxol #1 went fine, with no allergic reaction. It took three hours, but thanks to Benadryl, I slept through half of it. We scored a private treatment room, chicken salad sandwiches, and cookies—perks of treatment at the "Big House." I felt like Superwoman this morning and made our favorite raspberry muffins at 5:30 am for breakfast. Wednesday, I'm getting genetic counseling after my ($6,000) Neulasta shot. Are any more body parts destined for removal? Stay tuned…

MAY 27, 2006

Alas, the Superwoman euphoria is gone, replaced by a "hit by a truck" feeling. My legs feel like they're at mile 22 of a marathon. I have night sweats and tingling fingers and toes. How lovely. The effects of the Taxol are cumulative, so this could worsen each time, but there are only three treatments left! Today I did the cancer triathlon: rode my bike to volunteer at a local hospice race, walked with the dog to mail overdue thank you notes, and finally did laundry. Close examination will reveal the link between these activities and each triathlon leg. Looking forward to a beautiful weekend!

JUNE 13, 2006

Six down, two to go! After that, I get three weeks off, then it's six weeks of radiation treatments daily. That's my summer.

I don't feel sick like I did with Adriamycin and Cytoxin, but I'm very tired. While playing my horn for a concert, I felt extremely out of breath, unheard of for me. My oncologist enlightened me: "You ARE out of breath" due to depressed red blood counts preventing me from getting adequate oxygen.

The musical theme for Taxol is, "I feel it in my fingers, I feel it in my toes." Remember the Troggs? My fingers and toes are tingly and strange, and my toenails are weird and bluish. Any weak spots, like my 2005 Achilles tendonitis site, are painful.

When something was difficult in Oklahoma, they'd say, "That like to ate my lunch," as in "That calculus test was so hard, it ate my lunch." Extremely difficult things could "eat your lunch before lunch." Taxol is "eating my lunch before lunch." Fortunately, I'll soon be finished, ready to move on.

JULY 19, 2006

I've been busy with visitors, Andrea's graduation, and other things. On July 5th, I had my final chemotherapy treatment. I brought along homemade raspberry muffins for the nurses and staff to celebrate finishing. Directly afterward, we drove to the hospital so my PICC line could be removed by "qualified personnel." I was happy to see it go and immediately went for an, albeit slow, run. I've rejoined the gym and am lifting weights to get rid my "bat wings," a.k.a. flabby arms. Maria and I have started "get into shape" two-mile walk-jogs. She's preparing for cross country season, and I am just getting up and running. I've run twice with my Saturday morning group, managing six miles both times. I'm wearing my heart rate monitor to prevent me from overdoing it, which makes John very happy.

On July 6th, I saw the radiation oncologist and was mapped, tattooed, and calibrated for treatment. After a trial run this afternoon, treatment officially starts tomorrow. I was able to finagle being finished in time to take Andrea to college at the end of August. After this whirlwind, we're planning a mini-vacation before school starts and life goes on.

Before cancer, I held a hidden pride in being active and staying "in shape." My family had the good fortune to live in Norway for six years while my husband and I worked for Phillips Petroleum. The Norwegians place a high value on outdoor activity, healthy lifestyle, and family. Therefore, employers are expected to offer after-work corporate sports teams and outdoor activities. Because I held a part-time engineering job, the door to company-sponsored athletic teams, ski trips, mountain cabins, and weekly track and cross-country workouts was open to me. In 1996, I trained for the London marathon with my Norwegian running friends but, because my youngest daughter fell ill, I had to forego the group trip to run the race and take in the sights and sounds of London. Living the active lifestyle so valued by the Norwegians galvanized the concept that exercise can be a fun and social experience producing lifelong memories. After we moved back to the USA, I ran my first marathon in Tulsa in 1996, the year I turned forty. We then moved to Australia, where I put the Melbourne marathon on my radar. Unfortunately, allergies derailed my training.

We moved to Rochester, New York, in 1999 and I found the Goldrush runners, my current running and social companions. We meet every Saturday at 7:00 am with the option of "6 at 6," an extra six miles at 6:00 am for those building up for a marathon or just wanting to get home early. Rain, shine, snow, or ice, just like the postal service, nothing stops our weekly runs. With this group's encouragement and camaraderie, I qualified for and ran the Boston Marathon in 2004.

Achilles tendonitis prevented me from running my second "Boston" in 2005. I needed the rest of the year to recover, just in time to be diagnosed with cancer. My vow to run through treatment was shattered when my medi-port developed a serious infection, was removed, and replaced with a PICC line. Because running's repetitive arm movements could irritate and compromise the line, I was reduced to walking three miles a day with our golden retriever. When my PICC line was removed after my final chemo treatment in July, the first thing I did was go out for a "run." I began building up my strength and endurance and ran my first post-cancer half marathon in August, one week after finishing 5½ weeks of radiation.

A local trail run led me to a chance encounter with a local group called Journeys of Inspiration (JOI), a community of support for people affected by cancer. I joined the group and together we reached the summit of the 19,340 ft. Mt. Kilimanjaro in Tanzania on March 1, 2008. This was the culmination of a journey that brought together cancer survivors and others with loved ones affected by cancer. By climbing together, we were able to boost our courage, overcome challenges, and celebrate life. In addition, we raised more than $150,000 for the American Cancer Society.

After completing this challenge, I wasn't sure what to do next. I had returned to the race circuit in 2007 and have since completed eight marathons and eight triathlons. When JOI announced plans for a trek to Everest Base Camp in November 2010, my first thought was, "I'm going!" Once again, I needed a new goal, something special. Since my first biopsy was on December 28, 2005, the three-week Everest Base Camp trek qualifies as a celebration of five years of a great post-cancer life. My trekking companions and I hope to prove that, with luck and good medical care, survivors can lead active and productive lives. This trip will be particularly poignant, since two of my Kilimanjaro "families" have developed metastatic breast cancer in the last year. One is currently in hospice care, and I plan to climb to Everest Base Camp in her honor.

MY BIO

A registered professional engineer, Alison lives in Rochester, New York, with her husband John and daughters Andrea and Maria. Since cancer year 2006, she's completed seven marathons and seven triathlons. She has continued horn playing, woodcarving, and her other interests. She keeps cancer worries at bay but faces the music at each check-up and Breast Cancer Coalition event. Her biggest post-cancer challenge was summiting Tanzania's 19,340 ft. Mount Kilimanjaro in March 2008. She continues loving life and her family.

Section Three:
The Holy Spirit

The breast cancer journey often takes on the qualities of a spiritual quest. As the treatment of the disease strips all the unimportant matters from one's life, the spiritual life beckons anew, and faith is there as a lifeline to buoy the heart and lift the soul.

"God is to me that creative Force, behind and in the universe, who manifests Himself as energy, as life, as order, as beauty, as thought, as conscience, as love."

HENRY SLOANE COFFIN

"Every morning I spend fifteen minutes filling my mind full of God, and so there's no room left for worry thoughts."

HOWARD CHANDLER CHRISTY

"I know God will not give me anything I can't handle. I just wish that He didn't trust me so much."

MOTHER TERESA

12

A Cancer Journey...
Lord, Heal Me! (Ps. 6:2)

BY THERESA D. BRONTE

"Have pity on me, O Lord, for I am languishing; heal me, O Lord, for my body is in terror."
Book of Psalms, verse 3 of the Bible

MY DIAGNOSIS:

My cancer was classified Stage IIIA, invasive ductal carcinoma. Invasive! I didn't like the sound of that and for good reason. The tumor had spread to the lymph nodes. Surgery followed shortly after my diagnosis: a partial mastectomy plus the removal of 30 nodes, eight that were positive.

MY JOURNEY:

I am a 79-year-young grandmother who is still surprised to see white hair in the mirror, even though I've had it for years. Inside I feel much younger and still enjoy a good time with my friends and family. I have raised four beautiful children; the oldest and youngest are girls with twin boys in between. My oldest daughter passed on at the age of 27, just after completing her Master's program. She had been diagnosed with lupus as a child, and the medication she needed to control the symptoms later led to several heart attacks. It was a difficult time for us all.

When my youngest child entered junior high, I decided to return to teaching at age 47, since I had been pursuing a Masters degree and now had my certification. I spent 17 years teaching elementary school and later became a reading teacher. My husband and I were married for 48 years until his unexpected death in 2002. He retired from dentistry one year before I retired from teaching, which was a great advantage for me. He was a marvelous cook… no, I mean chef. I came home to a wonderful dinner every evening during that last year of school. Not only did the house smell great, but the presentation of the food and wine couldn't be beat. I was truly spoiled and loved it.

I also have five grandchildren who are the light of my life. We are very close, and their parents are very generous in sharing their lives with me. My family has been truly wonderful and supportive of me at this time. Whether bringing over a meal, taking me to the doctor, or just being comforting, they have been there for me. I am very proud of them.

I first started on this cancer journey after being diagnosed with a tumor in the right breast. I was truly surprised. I believed, illogically, that because my sister survived breast cancer in her early 50s, other members of my family would not contract the disease. How could I have gotten "the big C," when I felt so well and didn't feel discomfort in my body? Even the achiness of my arthritis had subsided.

In a mammogram the previous month, nothing abnormal had been detected. Three weeks later at my annual checkup, my internist detected the lump. My reaction to the diagnosis was mixed. I believed it at first and then I didn't. After all, the mammogram of three weeks before had come back negative. Two biopsies and several X-rays later confirmed that I did indeed have cancer.

This wasn't supposed to happen to me. But it did. I had cancer, and I was starting on this unwanted journey, learning about drugs and procedures unknown to me. This was completely different from what my sister had experienced 30 years before and a real eye-opener for me, something not within the normal scope of my reality.

When the doctors first diagnosed my disease, I was more surprised than anything. Now I began to worry and all the "ifs, ands, and buts" came to mind that I hadn't even considered before. My mortality came into a much sharper focus. How could I feel so good (following the surgery and immediate aftermath) and have such a dire diagnosis with nodes involved?

As my precarious journey continued, I went to the cancer center where I would receive both chemotherapy and radiation. You cannot imagine the peace and tranquility that greeted me from the first moment I walked in the door. All my fears and misconceptions about the treatment quickly faded away. Everything that I had dreaded before had now become "doable." The only thing that bothered me were the bouts of fatigue that came and went with the treatments, but even those concerns were erased by the love and compassion of the good people treating me. You couldn't help but feel positive in such a warm community.

I was very fortunate to have experienced no discomfort or illness during my treatments. Every effort was made by the doctors and nurses to prevent side effects, and I was the beneficiary of their great efforts. My treatments were spread out with longer periods in between treatments because of my "advanced age," and my caregivers' concerns about my tolerance for the medications. Time did not drag as I had feared it would. Before long, the 12 chemo and 28 radiation sessions were completed. I firmly believe that keeping a positive attitude and occupying time with favorite activities is definitely the way to proceed. I know not all women have the same reactions to the treatments or have the same results. Although my situation seemed so easy in comparison to others, it doesn't change the outcome.

I want to tell you a little about my friend and neighbor Kathy, who taught me an important lesson. She was a lovely woman with an infectious laugh, so full of life. She was almost young enough to be my daughter. I knew she had been diagnosed with breast cancer about two years before I was. Coincidentally, she and I went to the cancer center on the same day. We always had much to discuss about how we were feeling and the like. On the last day we saw each other there, she casually mentioned that she had had a setback, and that the cancer had spread to her brain. It was as if she was telling me that the sun was shining outside. She told it as it was, with no tears, just her own sweet self. What a brave woman! Through our little conversations, she always had been cheerful, never complaining about her illness. She was looking forward to the birth of her daughter's first child, whom she expected in April. Well, Kathy didn't make it. She died two weeks after our final conversation. Her memorial service was on a beautiful sunny winter day, just as she would have loved. She taught me that we have to take life as it comes and make every day count. This was and is a very important lesson.

I have not yet come to the end of my cancer journey, as I do not know the final outcome. At this point in time, my tests have come back negative, which is a great plus. I know that I have sounded a little blasé when I said I have had a relatively easy time, but things can change at a moment's notice. I do believe in the Lord God and in the power of prayer. I also know that no prayer goes unanswered, though the answer may not be exactly what we had asked for.

I had a dear Aunt Alice who lived to be 106 and never took a pill until she was 100. I have a ways to go to get there, but I'm sure going to try to come close. I have those five grandkids to watch grow up, and hopefully they can live in a world free of cancer. I have faith that I can attend my grandson's high school graduation, go to Lake Superior to visit my son and his wife this summer, and be able to follow through on plans for a trip to England in the fall. There are so many other things I wish to do before my time on Earth is spent. I can only leave it up to the Lord who can heal me. If that is not in the plan, so be it. When I think that I have already reached seventy-nine, I am amazed. I never thought I would be so old and yet still so young, all at the same time.

As I am writing this last bit in my journal, it is raining outdoors. It is that quiet, soft rain that is so good for the lawn after a long, cold winter. As I watch, I can already see the grass turning a brighter green. It is so good to see the crocuses and daffodils blooming. I know that life in general and my family in particular, are much more precious to me. My wish is that anyone facing a similar situation may experience what I did. The Lord has been good to me. Peace.

MY BIO

Theresa Bronte is a native of the Rochester area and has lived in Pittsford since 1966. She was married to Dr. Dominic Bronte, a well-known dentist in Rochester, for 48 years. She attended Nazareth College, where she received her B.A. and M.S. in Education. She taught remedial reading and math in the Gates Chili school system for eighteen years. Ms. Bronte has been retired since 1990 and spends her time with family, volunteers for the St. Louis Parish, and travels to Europe every year.

13

Stronger Now

BY JUDY WOOD

"The power of positive thinking is stronger in fighting disease than all of the technology of modern medicine."
Thomas W. Allen

MY DIAGNOSIS:

I was diagnosed with Stage 0 DCIS with microcalcifications in the duct in the breast.

MY JOURNEY:

This is not going to be easy, my story. As I wander back through my Day-Timer for 2008, it amazes me that I was able to accomplish everything that I did. It makes me tired, just to read it. Being a real estate broker is a wild and crazy business in itself. Being in the real estate business for yourself is insane! Looking back, I realize I had volunteered for too many committees and meetings. The church dinners and homemade pies: they have to be homemade in my book!

My mammogram was scheduled on a Monday in early May, both breasts this year. Don't forget to not wear deodorant. I had been going every six months for two-and-a-half years. The doctors were watching the left breast. I would have a mammogram on both breasts, then six months later, just on the left breast. Every six months there was something suspicious, but not really anything to worry about. I waited for the doctor to read the x-rays and come in to speak to me. She said there was a computer malfunction and that the views obtained could not be transmitted to the diagnostic console for assessment. Huh? She asked me to please re-schedule for another diagnostic mammogram within the week.

My work went on at a fast pace, as always, with phone calls to clients, banks, and mortgage specialists. I had scheduled several meetings that required my attendance. I had a haircut and gave a haircut to our son, Frank. You name it, I'd probably done it! There were dinners at church, pies to make, and Father's Day to celebrate. We even went to a wedding that Friday evening.

The following Monday, I went back for another mammogram. The doctor seemed to choose her words very carefully, telling me I needed further testing. She explained that the mammogram showed two separate groupings of microcalcifications, or tiny clusters of small calcium deposits in the right breast: one posterior at about 4 o'clock, and one centrally located. The numbers of these calcifications appeared to have increased since the last exam, six months before. In the past, these calcium deposits were there, but they had not clumped together. Now they had clustered together. She suggested that I see a radiologist for a stereotatic core needle biopsy. This is a mammographically guided breast biopsy. It is an excellent way to evaluate calcium deposits or tiny masses that are not visible with ultrasound.

Amazingly enough, for the next ten days, I again continued my hectic schedule. Three more haircuts were on the books for family members, which I love to do, and on the day before I had the biopsy, June 25, 2008, I took my granddaughter, Shannon, for her road test, and she passed!

Shannon was going to graduate from high school on Friday, June 27, 2008 at 7 pm. Our daughter Michelle, son-in-law Randy, and two grandchildren, Rebecca and Matthew, were to arrive from Virginia for the graduation at about 4 o'clock. We cut things a little close sometimes!

On Thursday, June 26, 2008 at 9:15 am, I was lying on the table while the doctors and nurses were attempting the stereotactic biopsy procedure. This is done with the patient lying face down with breasts hanging freely through an opening in the table. The table is then raised and the procedure is performed beneath the table using a specialized mammography unit used to produce diagnostic mammograms. The location of my cancer was in my right breast very close to my chest wall at about 3 to 4 o'clock.

Although the doctors and nurses made about fifteen or more attempts, they told me they just could not catch the area in the mammography unit. They wanted to try it a different way, by ultrasound and a core biopsy. The doctor said it would be very difficult to locate the area with ultrasound and actually hit the targeted area with the needle, but if I was willing to try, so were they. The only thing was, I hadn't been scheduled for an ultrasound machine that day, so my wait was four hours. The staff was very gracious, bringing me juice, crackers, and reading material. I may have even closed my eyes for a moment or two.

The machine finally became available, and the procedure came off without a hitch. One last bit of "torture" after all that: I had to have "one more mammogram" (which turned out to be three more) on that breast to make sure they hit the target! They had placed a tissue marker in the breast at the cancer site. The radiologist told me that since it was late in the day on Thursday, I probably wouldn't hear from them with the pathology results until Monday. "But," she said, "it doesn't look good."

It was Friday, June 27, 2008 at 2 pm, a warm day for June in Rochester, New York, when I received the phone call.

"I'm very sorry," she said, "You will need to see a surgeon. The diagnosis is DCIS, Ductal Carcinoma In Situ in the very early stage, Stage 0, microcalcifications in the duct in the right breast. You have breast cancer."

I remember saying thank you for the call. I did not cry. Is this what shock is? I have always handled fear by facing it head on! I am usually a fast thinker and act on impulse. My husband, Harry, came home about an hour later. The minute he walked in the door, he knew by the look on my face that I had received the call and what the results were. After 32 years of marriage, we can pretty much read each other. It's as if we are one, sometimes.

If it is possible, Harry and I have become closer since my diagnosis. We were already soul mates, but through our faith in God, we are even closer. I told him that in no uncertain terms were we going to tell anyone about this until after Shannon's graduation and her party on the 28th. Am I strong? Where does it come from? Being a mother, a grandmother, a daughter, a wife? Judy put on the smile and the attitude that Judy had to put on, for everyone else mattered more than this diagnosis on this day.

After the graduation celebration, I quietly asked all of our children: son Frank and his family, son Todd, daughter Michelle and her family, daughter Katie, and mom, to please stop back at the house, as I had something to tell them. I wanted to tell them something great, something wonderful, something exciting, something good, but… With God beside me, as I looked around the room at each of their faces, the faces of my family, my whole reason for being, I told them I had been diagnosed with breast cancer. Stillness, soft cries, questions I couldn't answer, louder cries. One by one, I went to them with hugs and murmurs that I just know God will heal me. I will be all right. We will get through this. It was the hardest thing I've ever had to do.

I had met with my surgeon the previous year, since things had been questionable for two-and-a-half years. The previous year, it was the left breast he had examined and at that time it was determined after a needle biopsy, that cancer was not present. He was quite surprised that I was back, and even more surprised that cancer was present in the right breast! With his expert knowledge and suggestions, and again, with God beside me, surgery for a lumpectomy was scheduled. I was sure that would be it. That would take care of it. The cancer would be gone.

Once more, that phone call came. The pathology report showed that the margins were not clean, there was cancer in the lobules, and atypical ductal hyperplasia was present. Basically, I am at high risk for recurrence.

I spent the next two months reading everything I could find about breast cancer. I attended seminars and support groups. I shared my story with everyone else who has been diagnosed with breast cancer, and listened to his or her story to learn all I could. During this time, a close male friend of my daughter passed away from breast cancer.

I found out that I knew virtually nothing about this horrible disease. Everyone is a little different. The major factor in my decision to have a bilateral mastectomy came from reading and studying my mammogram reports from the last two-and-a-half years. I addressed question after question to the health care professionals, my surgeon, radiologist, and friends. Why would I have another lumpectomy when the margins could still not be clean? Why would I not have both breasts off, when for two-and-a-half years, the doctors had been watching the left breast? Now, there is cancer in the right breast! The decision was crystal clear to me.

Harry and I took a ten-day vacation to Hatteras Island, a wonderful place to breathe and think and laugh and love. We came home with clear minds and a sense of peacefulness in our hearts, knowing that together, we had made the right choice.

My surgery was on October 29, 2008, and I have not looked back. I knew in my heart that it was the best decision for me, and I still believe that today, 18 months later. I had a right axillary sentinel lymph node biopsy; no metastatic carcinoma found in two lymph nodes. I had a bilateral mastectomy with no chemotherapy or additional medications recommended.

The prayers and support from our family and friends was overwhelming. Meals were brought in, along with beautiful flowers, gifts, and hundreds of cards. I also have found love and support from the Breast Cancer Coalition, where I continue to meet amazingly beautiful people, who, just like me, have been on and continue to be on, this journey. It doesn't stop.

I participated in The Pink Ribbon Walk last Mother's Day, where all of the money raised stays in Rochester, New York. My goal was $100, and I raised $1,000! This breast cancer journey is a long and winding road with bumps and potholes that we all will continue to walk every day. I believe we all have a Higher Being walking with us, giving us each day, one step at a time.

My faith has grown stronger since my diagnosis. I have learned how to pray. We have talks every day, God and I. He is a great listener and He gives me answers to all of my crazy questions. He teaches me patience, gives me strength, and is showing me how to live my life, this life He gave to me.

"I can do everything through Christ who gives me strength."

PHILIPPIANS 4:13

"Don't count the days, make the days count."

MUHAMMAD ALI.

MY BIO

I have been married to my best friend, Harry, for 34 years. We have two sons and two daughters, seven grandchildren, and five great-grandchildren. I am forever grateful to still have my mom, whose love, strength, and wisdom are with me every day. I am a real estate broker and love to dabble in oil painting, reading, and gardening.

14

Faith in God...
Dancing with Hope

BY JANET STAGER

"...A time to weep and a time to laugh, a time to mourn and a time to dance."
Ecclesiastes 3:4

MY DIAGNOSIS:

I was diagnosed with lobular carcinoma of the right breast, HER2 negative, estrogen positive.

MY JOURNEY:

My surgeon called to inform me that the biopsy from the lump excised the previous week was malignant. It was April 19, 2005, the exact day the previous year when I had been diagnosed with stomach cancer. My first thought was, "Does God have a sense of humor or what?" I just don't believe in coincidences.

The lump in my breast had been discovered the prior year during a routine gynecological check-up. My doctor thought it was just a granuloma and nothing to worry about. Several months later, after the stomach cancer diagnosis, the doctors also checked out an ovarian cyst (which had been identified in a CT scan prior to the stomach surgery) and declared both the breast lump and the ovarian cysts benign. Their main concern was the stomach.

After a partial gastrectomy, I was sent home "healthy." I have since learned that only a pathologist can definitively diagnose cancer.

At my next mammogram, the radiologist wisely referred me to my surgeon for a needle biopsy of the cyst, just to be sure. Given inconclusive pathologic results, the decision was made to "watch it" every few months. Every three months I went back to the surgeon, and he did another needle biopsy. In March 2005 at my next mammogram, the radiologist performed an ultrasound, concluded the lump had gotten a bit larger, and referred me immediately to my surgeon. He recommended that the lump be removed. He expected it to be benign. I found this all to be a bit of a bother, since I was busy living my life, dancing, and I really didn't have time to be in the hospital.

I think my surgeon was as surprised as I was to find the pathology of the lump to be malignant with positive margins. That finding was followed by a sentinel node biopsy procedure performed by my surgeon. We were able to co-ordinate with my OB/GYN to also remove my ovaries at the same time, "just to make sure they were OK." Thank God, the ovarian cyst was benign, BUT, surprise, three out of the eleven lymph nodes in the armpit were cancerous.

After having a second opinion from another oncologist, I began eight rounds of chemo (Cytoxin and Adriamycin and Taxotere) followed by a second excision to make sure the chemo had been successful. It wasn't.

Due to more positive margins, both the surgeon and oncologist recommended I have a mastectomy followed by six-plus weeks of radiation. The pathology of the mastectomy found those margins clear. The cancer was kept in check with Arimidex pills to hopefully keep any stray cancer cells from growing, since mine fed on estrogen. I stayed on this drug for three-and-one-half years.

The side effects of active chemo treatment were interesting. Besides the fatigue and muscle aches, which frustrated me, losing my hair was very difficult. Why is it that when you dye your hair, you are lucky if it doesn't begin to grow out by the time you get home, yet when you lose all your hair, after the treatment stops it takes forever to come back in! I hated losing my eyelashes and nasal hair too! Oncologists never mention those details.

Oh yes, God does have a sense of humor, as my hair finally grew in a beautiful shade of silver but very kinky curly. I had always had very fine, straight, mousey brown hair. This was quite the change. Since in my mind's eye, I had always seen myself as a brunette, it took a long time for me to recognize this stranger with the silver hair who was looking back at me in the mirror! When the oncology nurse helped me choose a wig, she brought me all their blonde wigs. Well, I've always had brown hair, but after years of highlighting it, it had gotten lighter and lighter. People always referred to me as a blonde, which I thought was just silly since in my mind I still saw brown. I wondered why the nurse looked at me funny when she then brought in all the brown wigs. When I saw the brown wigs I realized, "Oh my goodness, I HAVE BEEN a blonde." What a shock!

I did OK for the next three years. Life returned to normal, I was back working a full schedule, and life was wonderful again. I loved to swing dance. I met my partner there, and we danced a minimum of once or twice a week. I had also begun to work with a physical trainer, and after three years I was finding my muscles getting a bit more sore than normal. I attributed it to the fact that I HATE exercise. I have always been underweight and never "needed" to exercise for weight loss. When the trainer was with me I did well, but when exercising alone I would rush through the routines and frequently wasn't as precise as he wanted, so we attributed my discomfort to strained muscles.

Several months later, after a vigorous night of swing dancing, my back muscles began feeling very uncomfortable. I scheduled an appointment to see my internist, and his registered nurse practitioner (RNP) recommended a bone scan and CT. I am not one to rush into testing, but she said I could either do it then or wait a week for my routine oncology appointment where he would strongly suggest it. I relented and scheduled the tests on December 19th. She called me on the 22nd to say my bone scan and CT showed metastatic cancer in my bones and liver. Merry Christmas! I still believed that God was in control and I would do the next right thing.

Since the Arimidex had stopped working, I was put on a regimen of Faslodex. After three months, a CT showed that this wasn't working either, so I progressed to Xeloda pills. I was on this regimen for almost a year along with occasional chemo boosters to enhance its benefit. The nice thing about the Xeloda is that it doesn't have hair loss as a side effect, and fatigue was at a minimum, so we continued with our dancing. This combination of Xeloda and chemo boosters seemed to keep the cancer in check until March 2010, when my latest bone scan and CT showed continued growth in my bones and liver.

"Okay God, what is this all about? Are you calling me home

or do I still have work to do here? Which will it be, Heaven or Health?"

I had gotten involved with my church in creating a booklet on God and cancer. It is a testimony by cancer survivors on how they handled their illness with their faith life. This was a labor of love, and I was determined to complete this since I saw the potential of the booklet to reach many people whose lives have been affected by this awful disease. I actually cannot imagine going on this journey without God! My faith has grown tremendously through the cancer journey. I know I can rely on God to comfort and sustain me, to be my counselor and companion. When the pain gets too bad, He leads me to a place where I can find relief. I willingly take more pain medications now. This is from a person who NEVER took pills. (Instead they were just injecting drugs into my veins! How ironic.)

I have begun acupuncture and have found wonderful relief, not just from the pain, but from a slew of other side effects, including a severe case of nasal mucous which was so bad I would frequently wind up gagging from postnasal drip. When I reported this to the doctors and PA's, they looked down my throat and announced it wasn't sore (did I say it was sore?), insisting I was nauseous. I would explain that I wasn't nauseous, but gaggy. They just didn't get it. I have also grown tired of them saying, "I've never seen that side effect before!" Well, duh, you have now, so remember it! I have been wonderfully created, and my body does respond differently than the average person's. The doctors are finally beginning to understand this.

What is next? Well, I just do the next right thing, which for me is the next chemo drug, Ixempra. Unfortunately, we are out of options where I do not lose my hair, but being wiser now, I have just ordered a brunette wig with blonde highlights. I pray that this drug will work for as long as possible.

One of the hardest things I have to face is my children's fear. They are both medical professionals and know too much about where I am headed. My son is more stoic and clinical, but my daughter is more fragile. I can't tell you how often I woke up in the morning spitting out dirt because she had already buried me! I think she knows now that I am a lot stronger and can handle this with hope and courage.

Yes this cancer will probably get me in the end, but not today. I am living one day at a time, and after all, this is all that God gives us. He has a plan for me, and I wake up each morning and say, "Good morning God. What is it you have planned for me today?"

Dance is very important to me, and I am grateful that we are still dancing. I dance a bit more stiffly since I have more muscle aches, but I will keep dancing for as long as possible. It is an activity that is good for me and my partner.

I have learned from having cancer that you can't do it alone, and you had better have a sense of humor. As I have mentioned, I have a wonderful relationship with God, talking frequently with Him during the day. He keeps reminding me that "*I can do everything through Christ who gives me strength.*" (Philippians 4:13) He walked me through every phase of treatment and was present in the hands of my friends and family who saw me on my good and not-so-good days. Dear friends gave me a plaque reading: "*I get up, I walk, I fall down. Meanwhile, I keep dancing.*" I will continue dancing every chance I get!

To other women, my advice is this: be proactive regarding your own health. Ask questions, go for your annual checkups, do your breast self-exams. Don't be afraid of cancer. It isn't afraid of you, and early detection can save your life. Then you, like me, can go on dancing.

MY BIO

Born in Brooklyn, I grew up on Long Island and moved to Canandaigua in 1981. I have been a Registered Dental Hygienist for 40 years, and a Mary Kay Consultant for 30 years. I have two children, both Physicians Assistants. One lives in Boston and the other on Long Island. I currently live with my dance partner, Carroll, in Canandaigua.

MOMENTS OF TRUTH, GIFTS OF LOVE

JANET'S FINAL WEEK 1948 - 2010

After a valiant struggle, Janet Stager finally lost her battle with metastatic breast cancer on Monday, June 14, 2010. Continuous chemo treatments and stereotactic radiation failed to control the tumors growing in her liver. During her last week, she went into end-stage liver failure and her health deteriorated very quickly. On Sunday, the elders of her church gathered at her home to give her last communion and she was alert enough to participate. On Monday, she was in a near-coma, but could at least hear what was going on around her. A close friend called, so we held the phone next to her ear, and she definitely smiled a couple of times and was heard to faintly say, "Goodbye." She passed into the hands of God a couple hours later, surrounded by her family, a couple of close friends, and her pastor.

Written by her companion, Carroll Wilcox

15

Shining Bright and Reflecting Back

BY LAURA ROBERTACCIO

"Do you not know that you are the temple of God and that the Spirit of God dwells in you?"
1 Corinthians 3:16

The sun continues to shine down on me and gives me strength to live my days to the fullest. I can look back on my life with great confidence and know that I don't have any regrets for the way I have lived. If I can influence just one young woman to be an advocate for her own health, I feel as if I have completed part of my role here on earth.

MY DIAGNOSIS:

On July 3, 2004, I received a phone call from my breast surgeon oncologist that my breast core biopsy had come back positive for invasive lobular carcinoma. My next step was surgery to see how involved the cancer was and whether it had spread. A left-breast lumpectomy was performed on July 17, 2004. A tumor measuring 3.5 cm was found containing lobular carcinoma. The report read that the invasive carcinoma extended to anterior and inferior margins and was .1 cm to posterior margin. A full axillary dissection revealed that metastatic lobular carcinoma was found in 21 of 23 lymph nodes. There was also extension lobular carcinoma in situ extending to new margins. The analysis of the breast tumor was estrogen positive 90% and progesterone positive 10%. The tumor was HER2/neu negative. A mastectomy of the left breast followed three weeks after the lumpectomy, negative of any residual lobular carcinoma, but with surrounding lobular carcinoma in situ. The comprehensive BRCA1-BRCA2 Gene Sequence test results were negative. I was diagnosed with Stage IIIC breast cancer at age 28.

MY JOURNEY:

I was a very well rounded child growing up, the youngest of four. I grew up in a multi-cultural suburban neighborhood and had a best friend who lived on the same street. My father worked and my mother stayed home to raise their four children. My mother made homemade dinners practically every night. We never drank soda or ate junk food (except Super Bowl Sunday) and woke up every morning to Rice Krispies®, Corn Flakes, Wheaties®, or, if we were lucky, Cheerios®, maybe even Honey Nut Cheerios®. My mother always made us bring a packed lunch to school (which I really didn't mind), and dessert was fruit. So, point taken, I ate healthful meals! There was minimal television, so we played outside most of the time, jumping rope or riding bikes. We were raised Catholic and were a practicing family, making sure all sacraments were made on time. I even spent nearly six summers with my Catholic youth group on weekly retreats to Assateague Island, Maryland. Those retreats sparked my real relationship with God. I thank God for those opportunities today.

Those experiences helped keep me close to my internal spiritual being. I hope and pray a similar spiritual connection will happen for my children.

As a child, I was healthy in all aspects: mind, body, and soul. At least I thought I was, especially in comparison to so many other "challenged" teenagers that I knew at that time. I grew up loving the outdoors, and I was an avid and competitive runner for years. Unfortunately, when I was 18, I was bitten by a tick while having relations with a boyfriend outdoors. How was I to know at that time that there would be consequences to loving the outdoors? The tick bite was at the nape of my neck. I came across the tick one evening when I was running my fingers through my hair. It was still intact and engorged. Gross was an understatement. I pulled it out, and my doctor tested the tick, which came back negative for Lyme disease. Within that following year, I did become sick with an array of weird symptoms, from not being able to turn over and get out of bed in the morning to horrible changes with my vision. I finally tested positive for Lyme disease a year after the initial bite and was treated. Honestly, I truly believe that my immune system was altered greatly after getting Lyme disease.

The Lyme disease story continued a couple of years later when I was 21 and had lymph nodes removed from my right axillary (armpit) area. They were swollen and red, but no cancer was detected at that time. The doctors linked the irritation to my prior diagnosis of Lyme disease. I remained quite healthy for a number of years after the dissection of my lymph nodes. I moved on with my life, but that wasn't the end of my physical problems. In fact, it was only the beginning.

When I was 26, I started to notice that I wasn't feeling like myself. I felt as if I didn't even recognize myself while looking in the mirror. I was now a wife and the mother of two children, and I would blame my "new world" for not feeling like myself. I became completely forgetful of typical vocabulary words and where I placed things, losing everything from cooking utensils to car keys.

At first, I thought I was just going through a typical "mother syndrome." Then I started to have physical symptoms where I would get dizzy while I would go on walks or even out to the supermarket or shopping. It got so bad that I wasn't even walking straight in my own home anymore. This was pretty bad, considering I was taking care of my two- and four-year-old children. After completing a stress test, it was apparent that my blood pressure was dropping to extreme levels, such as 60/40. The doctors kept suggesting it was related to my Lyme disease, but I wasn't convinced. My blood work would always come back normal, so it was puzzling why I had such crazy symptoms with nothing to connect the dots.

In October 2003, after months and months of researching, seeing all sorts of specialists, and having many diagnostic tests done, I had emergency surgery for a microscopic rupturing appendix. At first, the doctors weren't even convinced that it was an appendicitis going on because I didn't have a temperature. Heads up to the medical field: some people don't always run fevers when their bodies are self-destructing! Well, after two days of excruciating pain, diarrhea, and vomiting, I had a CT scan that showed it was appendicitis. After surgery and four days in the hospital being pumped with antibiotics and fluids, I have to admit, I felt great. The doctors who were taking care of me before the surgery were confident that they could relate all my prior symptoms to a chronic appendicitis. Considering how good I felt after the surgery, I agreed with them. To tell the truth, I wanted an answer to all of the reasons why I hadn't felt well before, and I convinced myself to believe in the doctors—for a while anyway. I wound up feeling great for months after the surgery until the following spring, when I felt a lump on the left side of my breast.

On that "magic" night in May 2004, I entered my house after a long day. It was an evening just like every other, where I was glad to come home and relax. We had just come back from a family Communion party, which had turned out to be a fun day. I remember getting my two children off to bed and finally it was my turn to wrap myself into my cozy pajamas for the evening. As I took my bra off, my breasts felt heavy, as if I was getting my period. Now ladies, I know we all can relate. What woman has never had that feeling, right before menstruation, of our breasts feeling heavy and sore, like we could plow through a dairy farm knocking down the whole herd with just our breasts? Well, after I took my bra off, I cupped my breasts in my hands for some relief of the discomfort, when what to my wondering hands appeared—something quite unusual. Indeed, it was a lump on the outside of my left breast, near my armpit area.

My first reaction was literally, "What the fuck is this?" My husband was still working, so I didn't have anyone to consult. As soon as he came home, I showed him my lump.

"Isn't this weird?" I questioned him.

His response was "Uh, yeah, you need to check that out!"

I am not sure he knew how to react, but I wasn't too nervous. Inquisitive yes, but not nervous. Basically, I was thinking, "Wow, maybe this could be the reason why I haven't felt like myself for years." Although I was completely ignorant as to what my future held, my world changed from that day forward.

In August 2004, after undergoing a lumpectomy followed by a mastectomy, I was treated for breast cancer with the standard conventional chemotherapy with four rounds of Adriamycin/Cytoxan followed by four rounds of Taxol. In January 2005, after completing twelve weeks of chemotherapy, I began 28 days of radiation on my left side, from the middle of my neck down to the middle of my torso. My battle wounds remain today: three tattoo marks on my left side and a full mastectomy scar of about nine to ten inches with no reconstruction. I always tell my friends it's the prettiest mastectomy scar I have ever seen.

It took over a year after chemotherapy for me to feel "normal" again and to regain my strength and energy from the toxic medicine. My routine and daily tasks were completely exhausting for a long time. Even with the utmost support from my husband, family, and friends, it still took a long time for me to just feel like my "old" self and live day to day without pure exhaustion.

In June 2006, after a routine CT scan, I had a scare of the cancer spreading to my bones. After seeking three different opinions from various cancer institutions, I decided to have my ovaries removed, which enabled me to take different medicines because now I was menopausal. For me, I was okay living life with metastatic breast cancer because, after all, I was already considered metastatic when the breast cancer had spread to my lymph nodes with my initial diagnosis. This bone metastasis "thing" was not painful, and the medicine seemed to really be controlling everything... I thought.

In 2008, four years after my original diagnosis, I felt confident that maybe I was lucky enough to beat Stage III breast cancer. My bone metastasis was under control, to my knowledge, and I felt great. My children were now both in school, and I was energized with lots of time on my hands, so I decided to go back to school to become a nurse. Just when I felt comfortable with my disease, the cancer came back with a vengeance.

In December 2008, after a routine CT scan, over fifty tumors were found scattered within my liver, and bone metastasis was now covering my skeleton. I was shocked! I felt a little more tired than usual after going back to college and I had some recurring acid reflux, but never did I think the cancer had spread to my liver. I was scared, nervous, and hopeless, and I thought this was IT: death was knocking on my front door and calling my name. I wasn't ready to answer that call, though. This time I knew that I had to stop and look at my life with a different perspective, direction, and dream.

The day I received the phone call from my oncologist telling me that the cancer had spread to my liver, I didn't know how I was going to tell my children. My husband and I have been upfront and honest with our children on my medical situation all along. Seriously, how can a 9- and 7-year-old possibly comprehend what liver metastasis is when it's hard for an adult to grasp?

That snowy day, I decided to hold off on the despairing news and play with my children outside in the snow. We built a huge snowman with all the toppings: scarf, carrot nose, sticks for the arms, pine cones for the eyes, and even a dried hydrangea flower that blew in our direction when we were looking for a hat. It wound up being a beautiful snow woman! As we were playing, we found a dandelion bud growing up above the snow-covered lawn. I pointed it out to my daughter. We both thought, how is that possible? Imagine a flower having the strength to rise above the battle of winter and continue to grow, even through the struggle of winter's cold temperatures. I immediately thought that God was shining down on me and giving me hope that things would be okay.

The first time back to chemo I cried, walking down that hallway, knowing how awful the road ahead might turn. The dreadful thought of being on chemotherapy for the rest of my life was almost incomprehensible and still is at times. I knew how torturous the medicine would make me feel, and I was scared to think that the rest of my life might end up with me feeling like shit.

After spending weeks of laying my arms open to God and trying really hard to listen, I began to hear His words and remembered that budding dandelion standing tall above the snow on that December day. I needed to stand tall too. I put my faith into that little white budding dandelion. I realized that the dreams I made previously needed to change, and I needed to make new dreams with God. That is exactly what I did. I resumed my life with God, my husband, my two beautiful children, and the kick start of chemo all over again with a new attitude.

I started by deciding to treat my body as holy as I could. For me, it's very important what I put into this "temple," and how it is used and treated. I treat my body with the utmost respect, and if I fall off the wagon, I start fresh the next day. I keep positive people in my life, and for those who are more negative, I try to incorporate some spirituality into our conversations. I have completed the Lance Armstrong program at the YMCA for people surviving with cancer. For me, exercise is energetic, therapeutic, and powerfully "controlling" of my own body. I love riding my bike and strength training to complete my mind and body. For my soul, I have incorporated Eastern medicine with traditional conventional medicine. I get monthly massages from a comforting woman who seems to have magical hands. I receive acupuncture from an amazing woman who pours her heart and healing soul into mine to help "save me." I have become very involved with cancer support groups and continue to educate myself on cancer causes and preventive measures. I recently attended Confession for the first time in nearly 20 years, even though I have been a practicing Catholic my whole life. I felt completely liberated after that confession. Recently, I have even joined my church choir and am embarking on a clothing line for patients undergoing chemotherapy. In general, I feel that I have tried to become the most holy, spiritual, and best person I can be living with cancer.

MY BIO

I was born and raised in Wappingers Falls, New York. I graduated from the State University of New York at Fredonia with a Bachelor of Science in Music Therapy. I interned at the Center for Discovery in Harris, New York, for six months. I was able to experience music therapy at its best by working with adults and children who have disabilities or who are autistic. I am married to my best friend and soul mate, Andy. We have two compassionate, caring, and beautiful children: Zachary who is eleven, and Sarah who is nine. We all love spending time together biking, singing, playing games, and spending our summer vacations at Assateague Island, Maryland. We currently live in West Henrietta, New York, where we try to dodge the winters and love and enjoy the summers!

Contact: arobertaccio@rochester.rr.com

(16)

Surrender

BY EVE STRELLA-RIBSON

"If you knew who walked beside you at all times, you could never experience fear again."
A Course in Miracles

MY DIAGNOSIS:

I was diagnosed on July 11, 2007 with infiltrating ductal carcinoma ER/PR negative and HER2/neu negative (better known as a triple negative). A mammogram had revealed the tumor in my right breast. It was classified as a grade 3, 1.4 cm tumor that was surgically removed by way of a lumpectomy along with four lymph nodes removed. I was a Stage I and no cancer had traveled throughout my body. My prognosis was excellent as I underwent four rounds of Adriamycin and Cytoxan and 33 rounds of radiation. Then on the morning of May 4, 2009, I awoke with a headache that lasted the entire month. About two weeks into the headache, I started feeling dizzy and vomiting regularly. I was diagnosed with Stage IV metastasized breast cancer that had traveled to my brain and lungs.

MY JOURNEY:

When I'm in a group of people, I can't help but wonder how many of them have some form of cancer and are totally unaware of its presence in their bodies. After all, at least with my initial bout of breast cancer, I had felt no pain and had no symptoms, just a lump that I had found the morning of the mammogram. When I had found the lump, I immediately wrote it off as a knot of muscle due to the heavier amounts of clay I had been throwing on the wheel in my pottery studio.

When I was shown the mammogram films, I remember saying, "It looks like a golf ball," and thinking, "I don't play golf." The doctor wanted me to stay and have an ultrasound, so I did.

During the procedure, I looked over at the screen and saw what appeared to be a black hole. I quickly turned my head away as if not looking at it would make it non-existent. I realized that I was staring at the "beast"—the cancer—and it was staring right back at me. At that moment, I knew. At that moment, fear consumed every cell of my being. At that moment, I felt as if life as I had known it had come to an end and would never look or feel the same again. I returned to the doctor a few days later for a core biopsy. The news was confirmed a day later. It was what I had thought. It was cancer.

When you learn you have cancer, your entire world is changed; everything is turned upside down and inside out. Your priorities change immediately, your focus is diverted, and what was important one minute ago is no longer important at all. Lunch with the girls is quickly replaced by appointments with the doctors (surgeons and oncologists) and tests (scans and x-rays). These became my new priorities. I put my business on hold and concentrated all my energy on getting through this crisis and coming out the other side as a sane and whole person once more.

I've always been a very positive person, but I knew that remaining positive throughout this ordeal was going to be the challenge of my life. I asked my friends to send me as many jokes as possible. "Keep me laughing," I'd say. I have always built humor into every aspect of my life and this crisis was no exception to that. Humor has always taken the sharp edge off even the most extreme situations. When I hear others around me laughing, I feel more at ease. For example, right before going to the operating room for my lumpectomy, I was asked for the tenth time if I had taken anything by mouth after midnight. I answered with a straight face, "Nothing by mouth, but I did have a piece of chocolate cake rectally". The OR nurse laughed so hard that tears were running down her face.

Following my surgery, I had four rounds of Adriamycin and Cytoxan. When I was being infused, I was lovingly cared for by my "Chemo Sabe," a wonderful woman I knew from a healthcare facility in Rochester, New York, where we had both worked.

My husband Eddie and I had planned a trip to Hawaii for October 2007. The doctors worked very hard to get us there, but I would have needed an infusion the day before leaving and an another infusion the day after getting back. On top of that, my doctors wanted me to stay out of the sun and not to over-stress myself by doing too much. The chemo made me pretty sick, and I just couldn't envision myself sitting in the shade on the beach and feeling like I was going to die. We canceled the 2007 trip and went in October 2008. We spent an entire month on Maui and on the Big Island of Hawaii.

With the chemo behind me, I launched into 33 rounds of radiation delivered daily. When this was over, my treatment was finished and I finally had my life back. My energy level started to rise and within six months was once again extremely high. I was back to work taking on projects that challenged my skill set as an engineer, writer, keynote speaker, trainer, potter, and artist. Once more, I had life by the tail. I was hanging on for the ride, completely unaware of what was growing inside me once again. Sixteen months after my first bout, the breast cancer returned with a vengeance.

In April 2009, I noticed my energy level dropping slightly. Eddie would come home from work and find me sound asleep on the living room couch. The first week of May 2009, I started dealing with a headache on the right side of my head, just behind my ear. This lasted the entire month. I didn't think much of it until two weeks into the headache when I started feeling dizzy and vomiting on a regular basis. Since I had not thrown up since I was eight years old, I knew something wasn't right. Eddie wanted me to see the doctor, but I kept on saying, "It's only a headache. It will go away." The entire month of May, my health declined at an accelerating rate. I was shocked at how fast I went downhill and became disabled.

Tuesday, May 26, 2009, I went to my primary care physician's office. His schedule was full, but I was able to see his nurse practitioner. She thought the headache was due to a migraine and sent me to have an MRI first. That evening at 8:30 pm, I went for the MRI, and by 4:00 pm the next day, I received the phone call from my doctor. He informed me of the brain tumor and expressed how sorry he was. He had already sent all my information to the best neurosurgeon in Rochester, New York.

Two days later, I was in my neurosurgeon's office looking at the MRI results. It was clear to me why I had been so sick and was getting sicker. The tumor was 3.5 cm and highly suspect as metastasized breast cancer. Due to the size and swelling of the tumor, it was pressing against my brain stem. My neurosurgeon said that if I had waited ten days more, I'd have died. He talked to my oncologist to see if any other tests were needed before surgery.

Monday, June 1, 2009, I had the PET scan requested by my oncologist. This was a turning point for me. As the technician was ready to inject me, I asked him what was in the injection. "Radioactive glucose," he replied. Why glucose? Tumors have a high metabolism and the glucose (sugar) goes straight to the tumors. Then the radioactivity lights the tumor up. WOW! From that point on, I stopped drinking soda, cut refined sugar out of my life, and started reading the labels on all food items. Basically, I stopped feeding the cancer with refined sugar.

That evening my oncologist called me with more bad news. The cancer was also in my lungs. I was lying on the couch, and Eddie was sitting at my feet. We both heard the news over the speakerphone. I was devastated. Eddie was hugging my legs and weeping. I fell into a momentary depression and felt numb all over. At that moment, I knew my life was over. At that moment, everything around me felt altered. I was searching for the positive person within me to come forward and save me from drowning.

My brain surgery was scheduled for the next day. I knew I couldn't go into the OR depressed. Everything was happening so fast that I had no time to process anything. I came to the conclusion that there was nothing I could do. NOTHING! At that moment I realized that I had to surrender, not to the cancer, but to the surgeons and to God. I needed to put my life in their hands and have faith that all would be well. As I held my request up to the universe, I felt a calming that quickly led to a strong sense of peace and hope. I knew at that moment that God was at my side taking care of me, and that tomorrow in the OR, HE would be guiding the surgeon's hand.

That night I slept soundly and woke up the next morning refreshed and ready. The calm feeling of hopeful peace was still with me and as strong as the night before: no butterflies, no fear, no nervousness, no second thoughts. I knew I was going to make it, and that knowledge made me even stronger. My attitude was "Let's get this over with!"

I woke up from surgery feeling so grateful that I thanked God immediately for getting me through safe and sound. When Eddie walked into the room, I was never so happy to see his face as I was in that moment. I can only imagine how bad I must have looked to him, and yet his eyes were filled with love. Eddie was with me all the way. He was there for every appointment and hospital stay. He is my rock. There is no doubt that he is the best man alive, and I am extremely lucky to have him in my life. After all, he did not sign on for any of this or what might come in the future. I love him so.

During one of the visits from my neurosurgeon, I asked the doctor if the bone had been replaced in the back of my head. "No," he replied, "the muscle located at the base of the skull is very thick and will protect the brain." So, now I realize that I do have a hole in my head, and from this point on, when someone tells me, "You must have a hole in your head," I can't deny it! The same thing goes for the large numb spot on the right side of my head. So, when called a "numbskull," I have to own up to that as well.

Three weeks after brain surgery, I began ten rounds of full brain radiation. The following week, I had a port surgically implanted in preparation for the chemotherapy due to start the following week. The chemotherapy (Taxol) was for the breast cancer in my lungs. The infusions would be once a week for three weeks, followed by a week off. This cycle would continue for fifteen weeks. During these months, I would be recovering from the brain surgery and radiation treatments that followed. I was sleeping twelve to fifteen hours per day. My energy level was extremely low. Eddie and I ate out a lot because cooking was just too much for me to handle, and Eddie's sole culinary specialty was popcorn. I had no appetite. Chemo kills everything it touches, so my taste buds and sense of smell were pretty much gone. Everything tasted metallic. I altered my diet drastically. I've concluded that choosing what I eat and getting exercise are the only things over which I have control.

In November 2009, my oncologist put me on a break from chemo. I still had some specks of breast cancer in my lungs, but he felt it was time. A break from chemo is like a release from prison. About two-and-a-half weeks into my break, I realized that I felt really good and had lots of energy. My taste and sense of smell were back, and eating was once more a joy. This stopped me cold and forced the question, "Is this me, the real me?" It had been eight months since I felt normal, and now normal felt strange.

December 2009, during a follow-up MRI of my brain, a 5 mm tumor was found growing in the same area where I previously had the 3.5cm tumor. Because of the small size of the tumor, the doctors decided to perform stereotactic radiosurgery. This is a technique in which radiation is beamed from several directions (stereotactic) and radiates or cooks the tumor. It is the latest technology since gamma knife.

On January 11, 2010, I entered the hospital for the procedure. A C-scan was done and then a "halo," a metal frame, was attached to my head. This device was barbaric in every sense of the word. I jokingly referred to it as "disco bondage head gear." A local anesthetic was injected in the four areas where this device was to be bolted to my head. The doctors wanted my head absolutely immobile, and the halo was used for this very reason.

The initial installation of the halo was incorrect, and the fitting had to be totally redone. Having this done once was bad enough, but having it done twice was not a thrilling prospect. As the halo was taken off, blood started running down my face. The local anesthetic was injected into four new sites, and the disco bondage headgear was re-installed.

As the two doctors were bolting the halo in place, I asked them if they had ever had one of these put on them. They looked at me like I had three heads and said, "No."

I responded, "You need to go through this and see how it feels to the patient."

They just looked at one another with blank expressions on their faces.

After the halo was repositioned, I had an MRI that was then aligned with the C-scan for the critical accuracy necessary for the radio surgery. The radiation itself was painless and over very quickly. As a follow up, the doctors do an MRI about every two to three months, keeping a watchful eye on me to make sure that nothing new starts growing and that the 5 mm tumor is shrinking.

At this point, life is good and I am thankful to be alive. I am back on chemo and most likely will be on and off it for the rest of my life. I am surrounded by good friends who love me and make sure I know it every day. When you go through something like this, you really learn who your true friends are. My girlfriends are the greatest, and I am lucky to have them. There is nothing anyone can do but be supportive: send a card, send flowers, listen, and be there when you need them. Eddie is close by my side giving me all the love I could ever want. I've learned to surrender and fully place myself in others' hands, trusting that all will be well and that God will be by my side at all times.

MY BIO

Eve Strella-Ribson was born and raised in Pittsburgh, PA. She graduated from Kittanning High School, Kittanning, Pennsylvania, in 1969 and from Rochester Institute of Technology (RIT) in 1986 with a BS in Industrial Engineering. Eve presently lives in Pittsford, New York, with her husband Edward. She is CEO of Strella & Associates, a consulting, coaching, training, keynoting, team energizing, industrial engineering firm located in Pittsford, New York. She is a lecturer on many cruise lines as part of the onboard entertainment. She is a published author, having contributed to five books and having written numerous magazine articles for Stephen R. Covey, *Rochester Woman* and others. She also does pottery, sculpture, painting, photography, and stained glass design. Eve's other passions are astronomy and equestrian sport. She rode her horse, Mr. B, to national champion status in dressage. Together with her husband, Ed Ribson, she loves to explore the cosmos from their backyard observatory, Stardust.

17

Complete Surrender

BY LINDA MORREALE

"As I awaken within your heart, you will know the truth, that I am all."
Vida

MY DIAGNOSIS:

In-situ carcinoma in left breast.

Tumor: Grade 1, tumor necrosis minimal.

Tumor size: 3.0 cm.

Tumor distribution: discrete, single-mass tumor extended into globules and anterior margin and is 1.5 mm from the deep margin. One of 21 lymph nodes positive for isolated tumor cells. Estrogen and progesterone positive.

The tumor was grade 2 invasive at the time of surgery.

I believe without a doubt that a needle biopsy that bled out was responsible for the cancer's spreading and becoming invasive. My gut told me to leave the office and not get the biopsy. I didn't listen. That became my greatest fear. I am now learning to listen and obey my inner knowing versus the authorities of the world. Being still and quieting the mind will be an ongoing mission of mine.

MY JOURNEY:

My story starts with my annual OB/GYN check-up. My doctor found a lump in my left breast. The lump was a good size for my small breast. I wasn't one who did self-exams. Touching myself wasn't my idea of a good time, although I make a fairly successful living healing others through therapeutic massage, where the human touch can eliminate pain and suffering. Soon after my doctor's visit, I made an appointment with a breast clinic. My x-rays showed a mass, and they recommended a biopsy.

While the clinic was preparing me for the biopsy, I had a very strong urge to leave and not go through with it. My mind overrode this feeling. I needed to know if it was a dis-ease called cancer. Dis-ease is the state of the body not being in harmony with itself and God. Unfortunately, a young assistant in training, under the supervision of a well-known doctor, performed the biopsy. Incorrectly, I might add. Afterward, I was bleeding internally as well as externally. A compress was applied for 20 minutes to stop the bleeding. This was not good, and fear poured in. I left, wishing I had listened to my gut... or was it intuition?

Later that week, my doctor called me. I had just finished my last massage for that day. No one was around when I received the news. As she spoke, I started to feel numb, as if I had just been issued a death sentence. I gave myself time to process my feelings. I cried for about an hour before calling my two sisters. We all agreed not to tell my mother that her baby had cancer. I knew her heart couldn't bear the dreadful news. My sisters wanted to help with their ideas and opinions about my treatment, but I had my own way—to follow alternative medicine and God.

I asked my sisters to respect my decisions, even though they might disagree. I knew no one could say or do anything to make this go away, so I turned to God within me, for He is my refuge.

The strength of my faith was on trial. How strong were my commitments and convictions? Was my faith built on rock or was it built on sinking sand? Would I fall into the dark abyss of despair, or would I raise my mind and heart to God, my Father. I knew He would keep me in perfect peace, as He does for all whose mind is stayed on Him. Although the battle to keep my eye singularly on God was present every day, my thoughts were that I'm too busy helping others get well though massage therapy. I had no time to think about me. So when negative thoughts came, I would say to them, "Get thee behind me. I am not entertaining you today."

I would pray and make God the focus of my day. Then I heard a quiet, still inner voice. *"Be still and know that I am God."* This was my new mantra, which I now accepted and believed.

I asked God to cleanse me, for I had to stand before God naked, free of my own ideas and opinions. Like a child seeking a Father's love, I had to love everything for no other reason, but to love everyone and everything unconditionally.

A date for surgery was set. My journey turned toward a quest for information. I had never been computer-savvy, but I searched on the Internet for knowledge of treatments and therapy that could eliminate the need for surgery. I sought chiropractors, with their cancer-fighting herbs. I drove two hours to Ithaca, New York, to see an acupuncturist who brewed more herbs. In three months, I was saturated.

Then I heard friends talk about the body's pH levels being alkaline or acidic. They talked about cancers and other diseases. They said that if your pH is alkaline, sickness could not proliferate.

I investigated ways to reduce the acidity of my body, and found an answer. I started juicing. You know, that "fruit and vegetable thing."

It took almost a year to turn my pH from acidic to alkaline. Even then, I needed to continue juicing to remain alkaline. I began making fruit smoothies. Friends poked fun at me with my green and brownish smoothies, but I didn't care. For the next two years, vegetable juicing and smoothies were part of my daily routine, and I was loving it! I now love to juice fresh vegetables and feel really good with lots of energy.

I heard about a nurse in Canada who had cured people from cancer. They erected a statue to honor her work. I read more about her, and felt she was the real deal, so I began taking Essaic tea for several months, until the cost got to be about $100 a month.

It dawned on me that I was chasing every idea to help me fight cancer. I felt confused and bewildered. It was then that revelation met reality. I turned to God completely and surrendered. I knew that He created me and that He can re-create and make me whole for His will and purpose, for His honor and glory. With God being my only reality, I prayed in complete abandonment the night before my scheduled surgery. The most amazing moment of my life was about to happen. Six months of struggling was about to come to an end. Let me tell you the best story. All the struggle was nothing but my personal journey to experience God in me. That night before the surgery, I prayed like I'd never prayed before.

My prayers opened my heart and mind to receive a glimpse of God's love. His presence was known and felt throughout my whole being. Truly awesome. I was lifted into this all-consuming love which gave me the peace that surpassed all understanding.

I was not capable of achieving this with any self-efforts, only by surrendering myself to God. I experienced the joy of knowing that God revealed His love to me, and that He did not abandon me in my darkest hour. I know that God was present. I was not alone. I sought God with all my heart, mind, body, and soul. In return, I came to know the peace and joy of knowing Him as Divine Love.

The big day had arrived for my scheduled surgery. I had slept very peacefully the night before and continued to have my peace and joy. In the bigger scheme of everything, the surgery, God, and healing, I wondered whether I needed to have the surgery. As these thoughts coursed through my consciousness, the doctor's office called to move my surgery one hour earlier. What was going to come out of my mouth would determine my fate: I heard myself say I would be there. I remembered that I am not my breast, that I was so much more than my breast. They could have it, and I would be whole without it for my wholeness knows God.

My sisters came to take me to the hospital, and I was happy. Yeah, happy. The joy from the night before never left me. The sky was blue and the sun shining. You have to understand, it was January 31 in Rochester, New York, where the sun doesn't shine much, so you really have to have the Son in you to shine from the inside out.

That was my state on the day of my surgery. In my heart, I knew God loved me. Even the nurse who cared for me said she was a witness to my joy. After surgery, one sister took me home and my other sister stayed with me. I felt much loved that week.

Soon after surgery, I realized my underarm area was numb. I couldn't raise my arm fully. For a massage therapist, that was unacceptable. Mild panic set in, with doubts about whether I could continue in my vocation. I started physical therapy, which continued for three weeks. Then I decided to work on myself using acupressure and massage and made great progress. Within one month, I was back to work fulltime, and I built up my client list again.

My oncologist and surgeon were considering Tamoxifen, radiation, and chemotherapy because one of 21 lymph nodes tested positive. As they debated various options, their uncertainty shook my faith in the medical system. I have continually heard it suggested that radiation causes cancer, so I had to make yet another major decision.

I chose to trust God. I never did Tamoxifen, radiation, or chemotherapy. And here I am, writing my story for you. I recently celebrated my fifth anniversary, and I am still strong and cancer-free. I have peace. And He is still the joy of my life. I'm finally on a healthier diet for my body type, which is tall with a thin frame. I also have many food allergies that used to affect my body with aches and pains. Juicing is a quick way to get good nutrition with essential vitamins and minerals daily.

Thank you for letting me tell my story. It was good to remember that when my heart is troubled, God carries me, as long as I can completely surrender my all to Him through prayer and actions, to surrender all of me, so that His will be done. Knowing fully and believing that God is in control of my life was my moment of profound understanding: I, of myself, am nothing, and God is everything.

My journey through cancer was an exercise that strengthened my faith. Was I going to let this name—cancer—override the power and authority of God in my life? Or was God my only reality, as Creator of Heaven and Earth? I'm here to serve God. He's not here to serve me. Like the prodigal son, the return is our part. God will meet us halfway. He did this for me. He can do this for you, too.

MY BIO

Linda Morreale graduated from the Fingers Lakes School of Massage, Ithaca, New York, in 1999. Currently Linda is a practicing massage therapist and owner of Healing Energy in Penfield, New York. She spent several years working as a chiropractic assistant and did catering while going through school. She has worked as a carpenter's assistant to build her strength and endurance. She has also worked as a photographer and manager at a photo studio.

Section Four:
The Changing Spirit

Cancer can be a call to action, to look at one's life, and finally to be the you that was always inside you waiting to come out. It puts life into a different perspective and gives it a new meaning. Life after cancer can look and feel very different from life before, with an unexpected richness of experience and joy.

"One must lose one's life in order to find it."
ANNE MORROW LINDBERGH

"If you don't like something change it; if you can't change it, change the way you think about it."
MARY ENGELBREIT

"It is not necessary to change. Survival is not mandatory."
W. EDWARDS DEMING

18

Time for Tea and Me

BY WENDY WHITE-RYAN, M.D.

"A woman is like a teabag - you can't tell how strong she is until you put her in hot water."
Eleanor Roosevelt

MY DIAGNOSIS:

I was diagnosed with infiltrating ductal carcinoma, grade 2 with cancerization of lobules and calcifications, Stage IV, ER / PR positive and HER2/neu negative.

MY JOURNEY:

I have always had lumpy breasts and by the time I turned forty, I had already made several trips to the breast radiologists for various complaints. I had a baseline mammogram at around 37 years of age. Just two months after my fortieth birthday, I began feeling increasingly sick over three weeks, and within a couple of days noted lymph nodes swelling all over my body. I also found a tiny dimple on my right nipple. At first, no one at the radiologist's office seemed that concerned about it. The radiologist, however, having reviewed my films and history, felt that there was more to the tiny dimple. "You either have breast cancer or lymphoma, and I'm inclined to believe that it is breast cancer."

Thus began my whirlwind of tests. Results 24 hours after a core biopsy done that day showed that I did indeed have breast cancer. An MRI showed a question of involvement of the left breast as well as the right. Because of the swollen lymph nodes and the fact that I had noted trouble breathing when trying to climb hills, I was sent for staging films. A bone scan showed lesions throughout my spine and ribs. A CT scan revealed the disease had already spread to my lungs and liver. I was in the oncologist's office ten days after I first heard the words "breast cancer," and I started chemotherapy the very next day! This seemed to be an aggressive tumor—already Stage IV. The doctor was offering hope that aggressive chemotherapy would work.

I had been devastated when the radiologist had diagnosed breast cancer. I sat all alone in my car at the parking lot and sobbed for a while before I was able to call my husband. Somehow I made it home. We lay in each other's arms crying. He told me that he loved me and that we would get through this. Then he picked up the phone and started calling people, beginning with my sister. I wanted to have the comfort of family and friends, and yet part of me did not want to let people know that I had cancer. Scott made it easier by reaching them and then handing me the phone.

We saved our discussion of my illness with our children, Connor and Sarah, ages eight and five, until we had an idea of the full diagnosis and treatment. They both knew that Scott's father had died of cancer from smoking before they were even born, so we knew that this would be a concern. When we did sit with them, we explained that before I had breast cancer I was a young, healthy person who did not smoke, and it was very different from the cancer that their grandfather had. We discussed that the doctors and I were going to do everything in our power to fight this disease. I explained that I would lose my hair—and of course this is what bothered them the most.

I have to admit that the hair loss bothered me quite a bit too. Since I was old enough to gain control over the length of my hair, I wore it long. As a child, I had been scarred by a hairdresser who believed that a short haircut saved money. I thought that with short hair I looked like a boy. When I had my initial appointment with oncology and toured the chemotherapy infusion center where I would start the next day, the bubbly nurse who gave me an orientation looked at my mid-back-length hair and said, "You're going to want to get that cut. It will be too traumatic to have it fall out at that length."

My family all went with me that weekend to watch as I got my first page cut in decades. I was, and continue to be, absolutely amazed by the amount of love and support that my breast cancer diagnosis has brought forth in all realms of my life. One of my best friends from elementary school flew in from California to spend time with me and make sure that I had accepted Jesus as my Savior. She has since made me a very special devotional scrapbook. Friends from work, from residency training, other colleagues, my sister's friends, acquaintances, neighbors, and other people from all over have sent cards, many saying that they were praying for me or that they have added me to their prayer group at church. Food has shown up at our house or I have been invited out for meals. Friends have taken me for chemotherapy and the next day's injection to boost my white cell counts. My roommate from medical school calls frequently to follow my progress. I have been invited to join a book club and scrap-booking clubs. My friendships have actually flourished!

My husband and I have grown closer since the diagnosis of my cancer. He has been my advocate, support, and comfort. He has helped me through the emotional upheavals that have occurred within my family over the past few years, including the deaths of both of my parents. Mom and Dad had stressed the importance of taking care of me, even in their last days, and my sister continues to remind me of this. She and her husband have prepared meals for our freezer, as have my husband's siblings.

My children have supported me in their own ways—sitting on the bed to do their homework, snuggling with me to watch a movie, tucking me in, and reading me stories. My daughter has given me "spas" with backrubs and manicures or pedicures.

Fatigue has been frustrating. Early on, my sister pointed out that I now had time to read a particular series of books that her family loved. They had given us the first two or three books several years before. I started with these and zipped through them. Within days of telling my sister how much I was enjoying them, a box labeled "owl mail" arrived on our doorstep. I do a lot of reading and am in two book clubs. I also watch movies and television programs or, when I am able and weather permits, I try to get outside and get some fresh air. Most afternoons will find me napping.

Cancer has led me to make many healthy changes in my life. Prior to being diagnosed, I used to feel like I was not only "burning the candle at both ends," but also in the middle. I was having trouble sleeping at night. I would eat the many treats that were prevalent at work and subsequently was overweight. I tended to eat quickly, rather than savor meals. I did not exercise. I knew that

I couldn't keep going like that, but didn't know what to do—then wham—cancer came along and changed all of that and more.

I had been practicing as a full-time pediatrician in an inner city practice for nine years prior to my diagnosis. I loved my patients but not the reams of paperwork, administrative requirements, and governmental hoops that came with them. I was being asked to see more patients each day, and yet I felt that I was barely addressing the needs of the ones I was already seeing in the time that I had. I went into medicine to work with individuals, not to work on an assembly line. It was very disheartening. The day that I was diagnosed with cancer, I called the office to tell them that I wouldn't be in that day, and I didn't know when I would be able to return. I actually haven't been able to return. I do miss my patients and the true doctoring side of my position, but I am thankful that the rest of it has been left behind through my life changes.

Shortly after being diagnosed, I began using a sleep mask in order to help increase my melatonin levels. I switched to a water filter that removes not only chlorine, but a number of other chemicals as well. I got rid of the plastic food storage containers. I ended up losing a lot of weight, partly because I wasn't eating the extras at work and partly because I wasn't as hungry.

After I had finished with my traditional chemotherapy, I went to see an integrative oncologist in Illinois. There I was started on a special diet along with supplements that I need to help my body regain the strength lost from chemotherapy. This diet includes lots of whole grains and organic vegetables, limited fats, omega-3 rich fish but no other meat, no milk, and no refined sugar. Green tea is a staple in the diet.

My family has been supportive of my diet. My kids often taste my food and like it. My husband still prefers his more traditional American diet but has prepared and tried some of my dishes. He also tries to find restaurants where I will be able to enjoy a meal. At age six, my niece told her parents that she wanted to be a vegetarian, so now she and I share special dishes at family gatherings.

The integrative cancer center also encouraged me to incorporate regular exercise into my days through walking, stretching, and strengthening. Rebuilding the body and maintaining the spirit are important in treating cancer and turning it into more of a chronic disease. I try to remind myself that chronic diseases wax and wane. Whenever I get particularly negative thoughts, I write them into a black notebook. (I never have liked the idea of writing ugly thoughts in a pretty journal.) I frequently remind myself that there have been so many discoveries in just the past few years with regards to the treatment of breast cancer, and I know that there are many more developments in the pipeline.

I was stable following the initial chemotherapy treatments, an elective removal of my ovaries, and initiation of hormonal therapy in February 2006 that continued through August 2008. Then, despite rising tumor markers and otherwise stable scans, I had headaches and vomiting. A spinal tap led to a diagnosis of leptominigeal disease (recurrence of the breast cancer on the coverings of the brain and spinal cord). I had an Ommaya (a "port" between the skull and the spinal fluid in the brain) placed so that I could receive chemotherapy in the spinal fluid. In December 2008, the disease began stabilizing, and I was changed to an oral medication for the leptomeninges. December 2009 scans have shown only recurrences of the bony disease and my medications have been changed this January to all IV chemotherapy. When my hair fell out again this time, my almost-ten-year-old daughter told me, "Mom, you can't wear the old wigs. You don't look like mommy in them." Guess who got to help me pick out a new one.

Nowadays, I start each morning with at least two cups of green tea. I try to sip one of these while relaxing, watching squirrels and birds outdoors or dog, cats, and ferrets indoors. The antics of these critters bring smiles to my face. Laughter comes unexpectedly from moments with them, the same way as it does with my children.

I still recall when my daughter told me, "Mom, we bought you a breast cancer stamp postcard so that you can always remember that you had breast cancer." Yes, dear, I don't think I'll ever forget that I had breast cancer.

I thank God, The Great Physician, for His guidance in my healing and for giving wisdom to my healers. Through Him and my own strength with which He has blessed me through this, I see myself as well and whole, holding my grandchildren.

MY BIO

Wendy White-Ryan, M.D. received her B.A. from Mount Holyoke College and her M.D. from New York Medical College. She completed residency training in pediatrics at the University of Rochester Strong Memorial Hospital. She is currently living in Rochester, New York with her husband, two children, and multiple pets.

19

Open the Doors

BY MYRA MORGAN, M.D.

"What lies behind us and what lies before us are tiny matters compared to what lies within us."
Ralph Waldo Emerson

MY DIAGNOSIS:

My tumor was diagnosed by screening mammogram in April 2009. When the clinic called to inform me that I needed to come back in, I was sure the "abnormality" was due to too much coffee prior to my appointment, so I went cold turkey in anticipation of a clean follow-up exam. Unfortunately the abnormality consisted of microcalcifications, which were about 1 cm in diameter and persisted despite my lack of caffeine. The tumor was determined to be Stage 0 DCIS by biopsy.

I felt completely betrayed by my breast and opted for a mastectomy to remove the offending appendage. At the time of surgery in June, however, a 3 cm invasive ductal carcinoma was discovered (not seen by mammography nor felt by human hands) as well as a single positive lymph node (the sentinel). Axillary lymph node dissection was performed adding an additional two hours to my simple mastectomy and revealing 27 more negative lymph nodes. Now the tumor was considered Stage IIB, hormone receptor negative and HER2 positive. It was time for aggressive treatment. I had four rounds of Cytoxan and Adriamycin followed by twelve weekly doses of Taxol and Herceptin and 30 days of radiation. The Herceptin continued every three weeks for one year.

MY JOURNEY:

For me, getting breast cancer was almost a relief. Not that I was hoping to get it, but I always felt like my clock was ticking. This was especially true as I approached 44 years of age, the same age as my mother when she died of ovarian cancer. I was only eight at the time, an age when I felt like I was the center of the universe. With her death, my universe lost all gravity. I had no thought as to how her death affected anyone but me, not even how it affected her. I would feel sick to my stomach every time I saw a hospital or went to a medical clinic. As far as I was concerned, the doctors had failed to do their job properly by not saving her. As I internalized my feelings of loss over the years, I decided that I would have to avenge my mother by becoming a doctor, stopping this atrocity of taking mothers from their children. Well, that may be a little romanticized, but when I did enter medical school, I knew my mother would have been truly proud.

During my time as an intern and resident, however, I found that treating cancer patients was particularly difficult. It took a really special kind of person with compassion, perseverance, and stamina for heartbreak that I just didn't have. The medicines were toxic and the surgeries barbaric, while the outcomes remained unpredictable. Even as an adult, contemplating cancer brought such an overwhelming sense of dread that I had a hard time not conveying these feelings to patients and their families, not to mention the toll it would take on my own psyche. So instead of oncology, I specialized in infectious diseases, a discipline which comes with its own set of challenges, but often results in cures after only days to weeks!

Once I began my career, I also started my family. After having three children in the space of 17 months, I continued to work on a part-time basis. Unfortunately, medicine is not very conducive to part-time work. I found I was always being pulled between the clinic and home, and oftentimes it was my children who suffered.

One day my nanny failed to show up because of an ice storm. My physician husband had spent the night at the hospital and was still there, so I would need to stay home. Luckily, most of my clinic patients cancelled, but the clinic staff called in a panic because one new patient had shown up, insisting it was an emergency. I woke my sleeping children, bundled them up, and carried them (in two trips) across the slippery road to the neighbor, a stay-at-home father, who graciously took the screaming toddlers as I struggled to get my car out of the iced-over neighborhood. I finally arrived at work, only to be accosted by an abusive patient seeking narcotics. I felt used and angry, as well as guilty that I had inconvenienced my neighbor and terrified my children.

At that point, I began to reevaluate my priorities. As my children began to talk, I realized that what they wanted most was to have me at home, and as I thought about it, what I wanted most when I was a child was more time with my own mother. So in the process of a move (I don't think I could have done it if we stayed where I was already working), I quit work and dedicated my time to raising my children. Meanwhile, I was approaching the dreaded age 44.

I tried to stay healthy. I ate right, exercised, began screening mammograms early, and had yearly pelvic exams, PAP smears, and even pelvic ultrasounds. I considered genetic testing for the BRCA gene but didn't pursue it, because I didn't think I would do anything differently. Although I felt great, I had a creeping sense of dread that someday the big crab would catch up to me.

Sure enough, at age 44, I went for that fateful mammogram. I was actually surprised it was breast cancer, since I assumed I would get ovarian cancer like my mother and grandmother. No one else in the family had been diagnosed with breast cancer. Despite the horrible sinking feeling when I received the diagnosis, I also had an odd sense of relief, knowing breast cancer carries a much better prognosis than ovarian cancer. At that point, I finally had the genetic testing, only to find out I was actually negative for the BRCA (BReast CAncer) gene. It is still likely that my mother did carry the gene, because other members of my family have since tested positive. At least I know that particular genetic burden will not haunt my own children.

My months of treatment have been fairly uneventful, if you could call all of the expected side effects uneventful. I felt sick, gained weight, lost hair, learned to wear nail polish, and basically learned to be a patient.

My family and friends have been wonderfully supportive, even though my own dog growled at me when I came downstairs the day my hair fell out. I had dutifully bought a wig in anticipation of that day, but never got used to wearing it. It didn't help that on my first day out in public I got into a car accident. As I was rear ended, the wig flew off my head and landed on the headrest behind me. I was too distraught to notice, but my daughter looked over and started laughing. She said I looked like I had two heads. I could never wear that wig comfortably again, knowing it might just leave me out in the cold like that. Luckily, as fall approached, I could wear a stocking cap and scarf, and most people wouldn't notice or care. Hair is a funny thing because no matter how well you feel any particular day, when you look in the mirror the reflection betrays you. Curiously, I now have many new friends who have never known me with long hair, or any hair at all for that matter.

I can't imagine how scary it would be to embark on this journey without the prior medical knowledge that I had, but I still find exceptional strength in other women who have traveled the same path. Each of them is an inspiration to me, as well as to my children. We routinely see neighbors, friends, other mothers, teachers, or even strangers who have had breast cancer, and they offer us strength.

My children will say, "Look, Mom, there is a lady with your hairdo," and I know I am not alone. Even more inspiring are those you would never suspect, who have quietly resumed their lives and shaken all but the shadow of breast cancer in their past until they say, "I've been there." Someday, I will be one of these women.

Now that my treatment is almost over, I can again focus on remaining healthy. Resuming regular exercise has markedly improved my sense of well being and strength, due in part to the Live Strong program at the local YMCA, where cancer survivors of all types get together to support each other in their quest to continue to live active lives. Participating in fundraising events such as the Pink Ribbon Run also builds solidarity among breast cancer survivors and supporters. Just finishing the race is a great accomplishment, and you can't help being inspired by noting the incredibly fast times of some of the survivors.

Thanks to the many dedicated researchers, surgeons, and clinicians who face this battle daily with their patients, I know the odds are on my side. I understand the sacrifices they have made in order to fight this battle with me, and I am truly grateful. I am no longer looking over my shoulder, waiting for cancer to knock on my door. Instead, my doors now remain wide open, welcoming the future inside.

MY BIO

Myra Morgan is a retired physician and married mother of three who enjoys pottery, tennis, rowing, and reading. She is an active school volunteer, promoting science education and creativity. In the future she hopes to run faster, teach, and perhaps resume her medical career.

Section Five:
The Family Spirit

No book on breast cancer survivors would be complete without the perspective of family members who share the journey.

"Sisters never quite forgive each other for what happened when they were five."

PAM BROWN

"A sister is a gift to the heart, a friend to the spirit, a golden thread to the meaning of life."

ISADORA JAMES

"Of two sisters one is always the watcher, one the dancer."

LOUISE GLÜCK

A Sister's Story of Love and Support

BY KAREEN JOHNSTON-TUCKER

*"So many of my favorite stories begin with,
'One time, my sister and I…'"
Tina Neidlein*

On a sunny day in July 2007, I was sitting at my desk in Aberdeen, New Jersey, going over some bills that had to be paid. The phone rang, and as soon as I heard Eve's voice, I knew there was something wrong. Instead of her usual happy greeting, she said, "I found a lump in my breast while I was taking a shower this morning." She went on to say that she was on her way to have a mammogram. She sounded scared, which is very uncharacteristic of Eve, but I needed to sound positive for her, so my immediate response was, "It's probably nothing, but it is good that you are going to see your doctor anyway." I told her to call me and let me know what the doctor had to say.

When I got off the phone, I sat quietly, thinking about what we had discussed. We do have a family history of cancer, and breast cancer is certainly one of the types of cancer that has reared its ugly head. But I thought, "No, it isn't cancer. She will be her bouncy self when she calls back, all happy and relieved."

I said to God, "Nothing that bad could ever happen to Eve.

I love her. She has too many things left to do in this life, and for the first time in our lives we are on the same page in our sibling relationship." I told God that she was going to be fine, but thanks for the little reminder of just how much I do love her. But events were to turn out otherwise.

While I waited to hear from her, I found myself thinking of our relationship and our lives over the years. We had not always had the best relationship as sisters. It took us a lifetime to learn to accept each other "as we were," to accept the differences in our personalities, and to appreciate and celebrate who we were as individuals. This was not easy because we were both headstrong in our perception of life and of the choices and directions we each followed.

A major turning point for us came in 2003 when I was living in Newfoundland, Canada, with my husband and son. Quite suddenly, my husband announced that he wanted a separation. My storybook family dissolved, my son and I were on our own, and I was struggling to make sense of my life. Eve came to my rescue. She kept me focused through constant phone calls. She gave me support, encouragement, and love. I could not have pulled through that experience without her boundless energy and advice. One of our happiest times together was when she came to Newfoundland to visit my son and me. We laughed and cried, and we had fun. I thought I could never repay her for those precious words and moments of support, but I also knew I would somehow find a way, and as I reminisced on that afternoon in July 2007, I knew in my heart that moment had come.

When Eve called later that same day, she sounded shaken but seemed to already be in battle mode. I listened in shock as it sank in for me. She explained that her doctor had scheduled a biopsy. When the results came back positive, the surgery was scheduled. From that point, Eve's life took on a direction of its own.

The next few weeks became a blur of activity centered on ridding her body of the cancer. Eve approached this as she does everything in her life: head-on, full steam ahead, and you had better not get in her way. I immediately e-mailed a worldwide network of friends and asked them to pray for her. I kept them informed of her progress and passed on wishes from everyone, even from people who did not personally know her, but prayed for her health. By the summer of 2008, she had completed her chemo and radiation therapy. Eve was a survivor. She had beaten the cancer. End of story.

Unfortunately, that was not the case. Part two of Eve's story is brilliantly captured in this wonderful book, which not only shares her continuing saga, but also brings to the forefront the stories of many other remarkable women who are fighting the same battle, all from the Rochester, New York, area. Too often, when we are struggling through overwhelming situations in life, we think we are alone and that no one else could possibly understand what we have to face each day. These women are mothers, sisters, grandmothers, wives, girlfriends, friends, employers, and employees. They are not alone; they are part of a growing network of women who have to balance the life they had with the life they now must endure with noble candor, one day at a time. They all hold the prestigious rank of survivor. Through their stories, we gain insight into their personal struggles, triumphs, and setbacks.

My sister Eve has always been "the wind beneath my wings."

When she walks into a room, she is preceded by a glow. I call it her aura. She is the person laughing, smiling, and talking to everyone.

I remember the time she visited me in Newfoundland. Her plane arrived in St. John's very late, after midnight. As I waited anxiously for her to clear customs, I said to the woman standing next to me, "My sister is arriving from the United States, and she has such a bubbly personality that you will probably hear her before you see her." The woman just laughed.

About ten minutes later, we heard laughter coming from the direction of the passengers coming down the escalator, and the woman next to me said, "I'd be guessing that would be her," as she pointed at my sister who was coming down the escalator, laughing and chatting with someone she had met on the plane.

"Yep," I said, "that's my sister".

Eve leads through example, unselfishly sharing and giving of herself. When she first mentioned her idea of putting this book in motion, she was between rounds of chemotherapy. I am sure she had some idea of how draining an endeavor of this magnitude would be on her physically and mentally, but her energy and passion had been ignited by the thought of putting these stories out there to show others that they are not alone, that this is how it's done—dealing with, fighting, and becoming a survivor of breast cancer. Eve is my baby sister, but she is also my teacher, my mentor, and my hero. She is focused and ready to go where this fight takes her…and she is a winner.

MY BIO

Kareen Johnston-Tucker has worn many hats on her life's journey including Information Technology (programmer/ systems analyst, computer operator, data entry), substitute teacher (all subjects, all grades), teacher's aide working with autistic pre-school children, and fingerprint technician with the FBI. She served in the United States Marine Corps (Vietnam era), did extensive fundraising, and most recently is working in customer service with Vonage America. She has also lived in many places including: Maryland; Pennsylvania; Washington, DC; Virginia; North Carolina; New Jersey; Oahu, Hawaii; Ottawa; Ontario, Canada; and Newfoundland, Canada. She is a graduate of Monmouth University and holds a Black Belt in TaeKwonDo, which she earned at the age of 50. When asked what her greatest achievement has been, without hesitation she will respond, "that would be my work in progress: my son Spud, who is 19." Her downtime is spent enjoying life, one moment, one day at a time.

Afterword

BY EDWARD J. RIBSON

*"Faith is the bird that sings
when the dawn is still dark."*
Rabindranath Tagore

The personal histories in this book are as varied as the personalities of the contributors with their diverse backgrounds, distinctive writing styles, and unique perspectives. Nevertheless, many of these histories have touched upon common points. First is the seeming unreality of the initial diagnosis of breast cancer. In an instant, life has been overturned and redirected. Life seems to be in a state of free fall, over which the patient has little or no control. While some patients are stunned (for lack of a stronger word), others respond to learning of the diagnosis with a numbed sense of detachment. Then there is the dread of chemotherapy with hair loss and fatigue, the dread of feeling so sick that good health is no longer even a distant memory. And, for some, the dread of having to tell spouses, children, and parents is nearly as daunting. Looming over all of this like a thunderhead is uncertainty about the future.

These stories have shown us that breast cancer patients deal with two separate and opposing realities, each of which appears unreal in light of the other. The first reality is the patient's life, the life that she had forged for herself and had been living until learning of her diagnosis. That life consisted of family, friends, neighbors, perhaps a profession or job, leisure time activities, and good health. In an instant, the positive diagnosis of breast cancer shouldered all of that aside and replaced it with the new reality of diagnostic scans, consultations, and possible surgery. Seemingly endless chemotherapy and radiation treatments sapped the patient of energy so that her previous life seemed almost unimaginable. Even the taste of food became virtually impossible to recall.

This low point is where the virtues of faith, hope, and love enter the fray and, as the stories in this book have illustrated, transform breast cancer patients into breast cancer warriors. Faith, hope, and love are not independent virtues; they dovetail with each other. Warriors need faith in a power beyond themselves and faith in their medical treatment to allow them to hope that they can regain their previous lives or build better ones. And they fuel their hope with love for life and with love for those around them. The rekindled love of life is like a lens that brings passions into sharp focus: they want to run marathons again and to climb mountains, because life is their birthright, and because they want to spend every second achieving all that life makes possible.

For families, friends, and other supporters of breast cancer patients, these stories have been particularly revealing. The stories enable supporters to see themselves through the eyes of breast cancer warriors. Cancer—or any life-threatening disease— can be particularly difficult for the spouse, family, and friends of the patient. Those bound most closely in love to the patient also require faith and hope and the ability to focus moment-by-moment and day-by-day on the patient's needs without neglecting their own needs. The breast cancer warrior's journey back to health is a spiritual journey for supporters too.

Ultimately, the stories in this book have told us at least as much about life as they have about breast cancer. For while it is true that we value the eternal, we also value that which we perceive to be most ephemeral: the beauty of a butterfly's wing, an iris blooming in autumn, an aurora dancing and shimmering like a veil in the evening sky of spring, the sudden flash of a shooting star rending the predawn darkness for a second. The encounter with breast cancer makes us realize that, like all of these, our lives are unique and fleeting and therefore all the more precious. No longer can we take anything for granted. We rediscover the smell of freshly cut grass and learn to treasure each step of a walk around the block. This heightened focus on each moment of life and on the value of those we love most, is possibly the most priceless gift that breast cancer warriors and their loved ones gain from this journey.

Glossary

angiolymphatic – when there are signs that the cancer has invaded blood vessels or lymph vessels.

angioinvasion – referring to the presence of tumor emboli or tumor masses within blood vessels and / or lymphatic vessels.

angiovascular – a tumor that has an established blood supply. Cancers need a blood supply to obtain nutrition and grow.

Arimidex – a hormonal treatment in pill form from a class of drugs called aromatase inhibitors.

atyical ductal hyperplasia - abnormal cells in the breast's milk ducts.

autologious transplant reconstruction - of or relating to a graft in which the donor and recipient areas are in the same individual.

axillary lymph node dissection – the removal of the lymph nodes or glands from one or both armpits. These nodes can then be examined to determine if the cancer has spread.

bilateral mastectomy – having both breasts removed.

biopsy – removal of tissue for examination.

BRBC - a blood test for breast cancer and ovarian cancer that looks for changes or mutations in the BRCA1 and BRCA2 genes.

carcinoma – most cancers are carcinomas, cancer within the epithelial tissue (skin, glands, and lining of internal organs).

cm - centimeter

core biopsy – tissue removal by inserting a needle into the lump/tumor without surgery. This is a routine test.

DCIS – the abbreviation for ductal carcinoma in situ. This is a noninvasive form of breast cancer.

ductal – a type of tumor that presents in the mammary duct.

ER/PR negative – When both estrogen receptor and progesterone receptor are not sensitive to hormones.

ER/PR positive – When both estrogen receptor and progesterone receptor are sensitive to hormones.

estrogen negative – female sex hormone does not show up during a pathologist examination of a biopsy.

estrogen positive – female sex hormone shows up during a pathologist examinaton of a biopsy.

extranodal – a tumor that is outside of the lymph node.

granuloma - a nodule that forms when the immune system attempts to fend off and isolate an antigen. The antigen can be an infectious pathogen or a foreign body, but in many cases granulomas form without apparent cause in autoimmune disorders.

HER2 or HER2/neu – a protein that is tested for by the pathologist following a biopsy. If positive, these cancers tend to be much more aggressive and fast growing.

hormone receptor positive – a location on a tumor at which either estrogen or progesterone molecules can attach; the presence of hormone receptors means a tumor depends on hormones to grow.

in situ – a term meaning "in position" or "in its place;" a breast cancer that has not spread through the wall of the milk duct or lobe where it originated.

intraductal – where the tumor or lump is located in the duct. These can be malignant or benign.

lesion – an abnormal change in structure of an organ due to disease.

lobe – one of the fifteen to twenty rounded divisions in each breast; the part of the breast in which milk is produced.

lobular – one of several small components of a lobe.

lobular carcinoma in situ – abnormal cells within the lobule that don't form lumps. They can serve as a marker of future cancer risk.

luminal – sensitive to hormones and slower-growing.

luminal necrosis - death of tissue in the inner open space or cavity of an organ or vessel.

lymph nodes – glands found throughout the body. These defend against invaders such as bacteria, and are generally examined and sometimes removed from the armpit during surgery. Cancer can spread from the location of the lymph nodes.

lymphodema – swelling of the arm can follow surgery to the lymph nodes under the arm. The swelling can be temporary or permanent and can occur immediately or any time later.

malignant – the medical term for something that is cancerous.

mammogram – an x-ray to image breast tissue.

margins – the outermost edge of the tissue under the pathologist's microscope. If clear, no cancer cells were found on the margins. If not clear, margins show cancer cells, and the surgeon may have to remove more tissue to get a clear margin.

mastectomy – the removal of a breast.

metastasis – the spread of cancer to other organs in the body.

microcalcification – tiny calcifications in the breast tissue. These are generally seen on a mammogram. When in a cluster, they can be a sign of ductal carcinoma in situ.

mm - millimeter

necrosis – dead tissue.

non-encapsulated – to not be enclosed in a gelatinous or membranous envelope.

nuclear grade – a system of classifying tumors that goes from high grade to low grade. Grade 1 is the least aggressive, while Grade 3 is the most aggressive type of tumor. The numbers assigned by the pathologist helps the physician make treatment decisions.

oncologist – the doctors who specialize in cancer study and treatment.

oncology – the branch of medicine that deals with tumors, including study of their development, diagnosis, treatment, and prevention..

progesterone negative – a steroid hormone produced in the ovaries that does not show up during the pathologist exam of a biopsy.

progesterone positive – a steroid hormone produced in the ovaries that does show up during the pathologist exam of a biopsy.

situ – a tumor that has not spread beyond the place where it originally developed.

seeds of radiation – a form of radiation therapy.

sentinel node dissection / biopsy – a surgical technique where a limited number of lymph nodes are removed from the armpit to determine if any breast cancer has spread.

Stage – measurement used to determine if the cancer has spread. Stages go from 0 to IV with IV being the most serious.

- **Stage 0** - there are 2 types of stage 0 breast carcinoma in situ: ductal carcinoma in situ (DCIS) and lobular carcinoma in situ (LCIS).

  DCIS is a noninvasive condition in which abnormal cells are found in the lining of a breast duct (a tube that carries milk to the nipple). The abnormal cells have not spread outside the duct to other tissues in the breast.

  LCIS is a condition in which abnormal cells are found in the lobules (small sections of tissue involved with making milk) of the breast.

- **Stage I** – the tumor is confined to a single site of the breast and it is no larger than 2 centimeters.

- **Stage IIA** – no tumor is found in the breast, but is found in the lymph nodes under the arm.

  Tumor is no larger than 2 centimeters and has spread to lymph nodes under the arm.

  Tumor is between 2 and 5 centimeters and has spread to lymph nodes under the arm.

- **Stage IIB** – either the tumor is between 2 and 5 cm or larger than 5 cm.

- **Stage IIIA** – no tumor is found in the breast, but cancer has spread to the lymph nodes near the breastbone and is between 2 and larger than 5 cm.

- **Stage IIIB** – the tumor is of any size and has spread to the chest wall.

- **Stage IIIC** – there may be no cancer in the breast or the tumor may be of any size and has spread to the chest wall and other lymph nodes.

- **Stage IV** – cancer has spread to other sites in the body, such as the liver, lungs, bones, or brain.

TAC – Taxol, Adriamycin, and Cytoxan, a common combination of chemotherapy drugs given for breast cancer.

tamoxifen – taken in pill form that blocks estrogen and progesterone receptors.

triple negative – when the HER2/neu, ER, and PR are all negative.

ultrasound – an imaging technique using sound waves to detect abnormalities.

unilateral mastectomy – having one breast removed.

Message from the Author

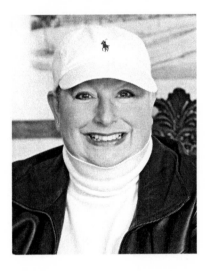

I want to take this opportunity to thank each and every one of you for purchasing our book, *Moments of Truth, Gifts of Love*. This book is for all who are dealing with aspects of breast cancer: caregivers, supporters, sisters, brothers, and other family members, all those touched by this horrible disease. We can only hope that what you take away from our stories, is a renewed sense of community and spirit. God Bless you.

Eve Strella-Ribson

estrella@strellaandassociates.com
www.strellaandassociates.com
www.linkedin.com/pub/2/978/294

LaVergne, TN USA
28 February 2011
218309LV00001B/8/P